101 Miracles
of
Natural Healing

Luke Chan

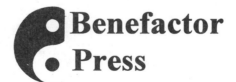

**Benefactor
Press**

To reduce the risk of injury, consult your doctor before beginning this or any exercise program. The instructions and advice presented are in no way intended as a substitute for medical counseling. The Author, Producers, Participants and Distributors of this book disclaim any liability or loss in connection with the exercise and advice herein.

Special Thanks to Dr. Pang

Founder and Director of Huaxia Zhineng Qigong Center.

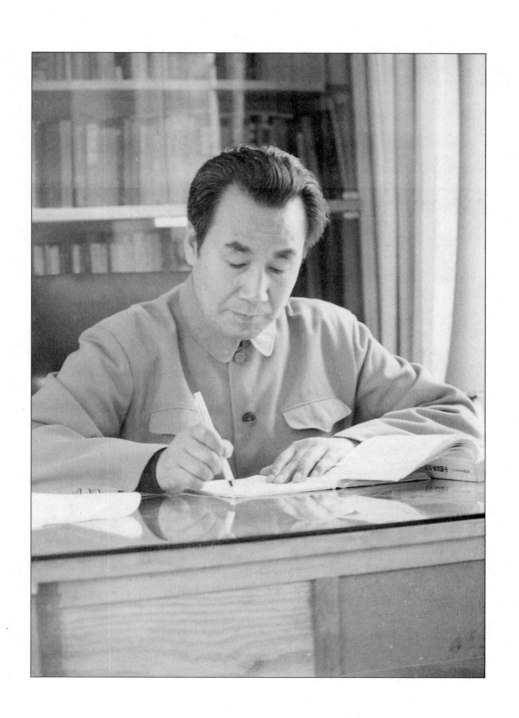

Acknowledgments:

I would like to thank Yu Lao-shi, the chief instructor of the Chi-Lel Academy, who arranged my staying in the Center and introduced me to various people for interviews.

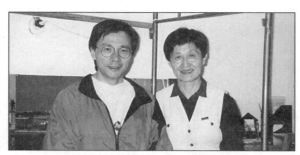

The author and Yu Lao-shi

I would also like to thank the teachers whose inspirational stories have changed my life for the better.

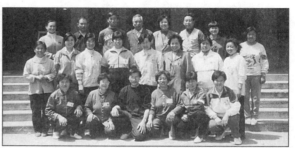

The author and the teachers

I would like to express my appreciation to the instructor trainees who sacrificed their practicing time to be interviewed.

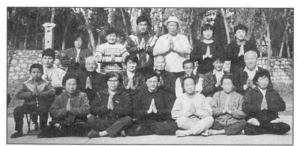

The author and the instructor trainees

I am grateful to the students who shared their stories. They sacrificed their afternoon resting time to pose for the adjacent group picture.

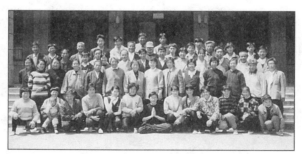

The author and the students

Also I would like to take this opportunity to thank: Teacher Leung, the photographer who captured the joy of the interviewees in her pictures; Teacher Hu Yi-sun for introducing Yu Lao-shi to me; all the teachers who arranged interviews for me; my editors John Goodell and Beth Franks; the book cover designer Pat Brooks; and my brother Frank Chan for his advice.

IV

Foreword:

I was stunned when I videotaped the ultrasound image of a cancerous tumor as it was being "removed" naturally, under the supervision of doctors, by Chi Lel teachers in China. I immediately felt that the self-healing art of Chi Lel must be a new frontier in fighting disease which everyone should know about.

Upon returning to the United States, I told many people about it, but most of them were skeptical, saying, "I haven't seen it on TV." So I called all the TV stations in my local area to tell them the good news. Only one reporter expressed any interest, and she stipulated that only if I had a doctor to comment on the footage would she consider looking at it. I called a number of doctors, but none were interested.

I thought maybe people weren't getting excited about Chi Lel because they had never heard of it, I decided to collect my interviews with recovered patients into a book. After finishing my manuscript, I gave it to my editor for review and later received a call.

"I like your stories, but...," my editor hesitated.

"Yes?"

"They are *truly* incredible."

"You don't believe them, do you?"

"Of course I do, but it's the average American I'm thinking about. They might be turned off by these miracles. You want to sell books, don't you?"

"Well, what's your advice?"

"You might want to tone them down."

As our conversation ended I felt unsure. Should I alter these interviews to make them seem more reasonable?

Then I recalled the emotion of a cancer patient who had been waiting three years to die because there wasn't any cure for his bladder cancer and who finally, with the help of Chi Lel, was given a fighting chance to recover and live. And I thought of a woman who, when being told by doctors that she was just too old for any treatment, refused to give up and fought her deadly disease with Chi Lel and finally survived to tell her story. Then there was the lady who had secretly practiced Chi Lel at home for two years because she was afraid of being ridiculed for believing in miracles, and who, when she finally went to a group practice, was embraced and "welcomed home." How could I deny these stories of human triumph over suffering?

To change these accounts to suit average beliefs would be a denial of encouragement and hope to those who truly need it. So the stories in this book remain exactly as they were told to me. Furthermore, I will endeavor to compile a sequel—of miracles involving Americans who've had the courage to try and triumph with the help of Chi Lel..

The World's Largest Medicineless Hospital

The Huaxia Zhineng Qigong Clinic & Training Center, simply known as the Center, normally has more than four thousand people living there, including doctors, patients, Chi-Lel teachers, trainees, and support personnel. The Center was established in November 1988 in the city of Zigachong and later, in February 1992, relocated to its present address, an old navy hospital in the city of Qinhuangdao, five hours by train from Beijing. It is directed by its founder, Dr. Pang Ming, a qigong grandmaster and physician trained in both Western and Chinese traditional medicine.

This hospital is the largest of its kind in China. The Center avoids medicines and special diets

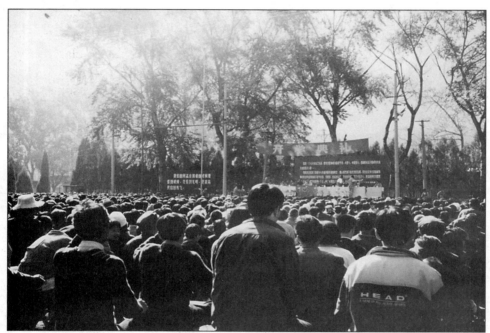

During the first day of training, students gather for instructions.

in favor of exercise, love, and life energy, or chi. It is a nonprofit organization and is recognized by the Chinese government as a legitimate clinic. Over the years, the Center has treated more than 180 diseases, with an overall success rate of 95 percent.

In 1995, I spent the entire month of May living at the Center, observing firsthand how the hospital operates and interviewing more than one hundred people who have miraculously recovered from "incurable" diseases such as cancer, diabetes, arthritis, deafness, coronary disease, paralysis, and systemic lupus. Many times I was moved to tears while listening to these accounts of heroic struggle against disease. One mother told me that she was so weak that she couldn't even pick up a kitchen knife to kill herself, and so attempted to end her life by not eating. But when her six-year-old son tried to spoon-feed her a bowl of milk while her eleven-year-old held a towel to wipe up any spills, she decided to live at any cost. Since doctors couldn't help her, she turned to Chi Lel and, against all odds, recovered. She is now a teacher at the Center.

Chi Lel, the method employed in the Center, was developed by Dr. Pang. The method is based on the 5,000-year-old concept of qigong (chigong, chi kung) as well as modern medical knowledge. Dr. Pang, reverently known as Lao-shi, the Teacher, has written more than nine books on Chi Lel.

When a patient enters the hospital, he or she is diagnosed by a doctor, and then assigned to a class of fifty or so people for a 24-day treatment period. Patients spend most of their time practicing Chi Lel, usually eight hours a day, without distractions such as television, newspapers, and telephone. Those who can stand up practice standing; those who can sit practice in their chairs; and those who can't move practice in their beds.

The Center has more than 600 staff members, including twenty-six Western-trained doctors. Since no medicine is prescribed, there aren't any pharmacists. Doctors, who prefer to be called teachers, play only a minor role in this special hospital. Occasionally, they are called upon to attend emergency cases. Their main function is to diagnose patients when they come in to register and again after each 24-day training period. Their diagnoses are classified into four categories for statistical purposes.

1. Cured: Symptoms disappear and appropriate instruments (e.g., EKG, ultrasound, X-ray, CT, and so on) register normal.

2. Very Effective: Symptoms almost disappear and instruments show great improvement.

3. Effective: Noticeable improvements; student can eat, sleep, and feel good.

4. Ineffective: No change or even worse.

According to <u>A Summary of Zhineng Qigong's Healing Effects on Chronic Diseases</u>, published by the Center in 1991, data on 7,936 patients showed an overall effective healing rate of 94.96 percent. This represents 15.20 percent cured, 37.68 percent very effective, and 42.09 percent effective.

The Center recently tried a new way of demonstrating the effectiveness of chi for treating cancer. I witnessed a cancer patient being treated by four Chi-Lel teachers while the patient's bladder cancer was viewed on the screen of an ultrasound machine monitored by two doctors. The cancer literally disappeared in front of my eyes in less than a minute as the teachers emitted chi into the patient, dissolving the cancer! In fact, I videotaped this incredible event. Ten days later, I asked the doctors to double-check if the patient's tumor was gone. The doctors put the same patient's bladder on-screen again and we saw no trace of cancer. Later I was told that a major German TV crew, visiting the Center a week before, had successfully videotaped the same process with other cancer patients

Despite its amazing success at healing, the Center is little known even in China because of its policy of not advertising in newspapers or magazines. However, the Center is well known among an estimated eight million Chi-Lel practitioners. Through word of mouth, thousands of people from all over China are coming to the Center every month. Indeed, Chi Lel has a great number of followers and the Center is the brain of this vast network.

At the Center, no matter how sick a person is, he or she is still addressed as a "student" never "patient." Why? Because students are learning an art, the goal of which is to heal oneself, unlike patients, who primarily rely on doctors. Therefore no doctor-patient relationships exist.

Tuition for the 24-days treatment program is only one hundred yuan (about twelve dollars). Including room and board, students can spend as little as six hundred yuan (about seventy dollars) per month! Probably the most inexpensive hospital in the world, the Center is truly a nonprofit organization. Yet it runs as an independent, self-sufficient organization, without any help from the government or private foundations.

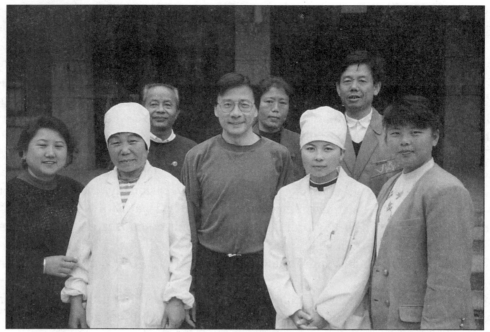

The author and two doctors pose with students whose tumors were removed by Chi-Lel teachers.

How do they operate so efficiently? Because many of the doctors, Chi-Lel teachers, and support personnel are former students who have recovered from serious illnesses themselves and have now returned voluntarily to serve the sick, with very little pay. Teachers play the roles of doctor, nurse, social worker, cheerleader, parent, friend, brother, and sister. Their effectiveness is measured by the healing rate of their students.

Another reason for the Center's effective but low-budget operation is that it uses group therapy. Students live in groups of four, eight, or sixteen persons per room. By living in groups, students develop a cooperative spirit of caring and love toward each other. Many of those I interviewed had been rejected by their former hospitals as incurable, and, thus regarded the Center as their last hope. As though sailing on the same boat in the ocean, students bond together against their common enemy—disease.

Just as hospitals associate with medical schools to train young people to enter the medical profession, the Center also has Chi-Lel schools to train Chi-Lel professionals. There is a Zhineng Qigong Academy as well as one-month and three-month instructor training programs. The Academy, established in 1992, has a two-year training program for young men and women under the age of thirty who have the minimum of a high-school education. The one-month and three-month instructor training programs are for anyone interested in Chi Lel. I was told that there are typically more than a thousand students in both schools.

In addition, just as prestigious hospitals have research programs, the Center has many ongoing research projects both on site and at different university campuses around the country. When I requested the person in charge, a retired college professor, to show me some published papers, he gave me two volumes of experiment data, as thick as a telephone book!

Besides doctors, teachers, and students, there are hundreds of support personnel working in the office, cafeteria, bookstore, and so on. All of them are Chi-Lel adherents who practice Chi Lel together in the morning and in the evening, about three hours a day. As they say, it is not just a job—it is a Chi-Lel job.

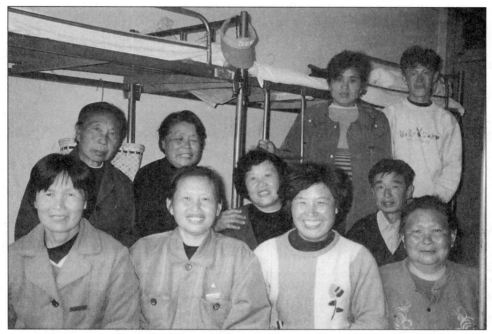

Students in their living quarters

The Center is open only ten months a year because there is no heat in the rooms during winter. The Center has been planning to build a Chi-Lel City, with better facilities, to accommodate the ever-increasing number of students, including Americans and others coming from abroad.

I asked the founder, Lao-shi, why he didn't promote Chi Lel to the world sooner. He replied that many people need proof of whether chi works or not. So instead of arguing with others, he preferred to work solidly by treating patients and collecting valuable data. As a result, tens of thousands of documented cases over a period of eight years have been collected and, "Now we are ready. Please tell the world that we exist and Chi Lel can benefit mankind."

CONTENTS

Acknowledgments   *IV*
Foreword   *V*
The World's Largest Medicineless Hospital   *VI*

Part One: The Interviews

Introduction to the Interviews   *2*

1. **If I Live I'll Repay Every Penny I Owe You**   *4*
2. **A New Life**   *6*
3. **What Miracle Drug from the West Have You Taken?**   *7*
4. **I Want to Live—I Have Three Young Children at Home**   *8*
5. **Being Deaf is a Horrible Thing**   *9*
6. **I Would Do Anything If Only I Could Stay Here**   *10*
7. **The Taming of the Shrew**   *11*
8. **An Ultrasound Specialist**   *12*
9. **Military Man Ordered Daughter to Go**   *13*
10. **I Have Returned**   *14*
11. **Double Happiness**   *15*
12. **Thank Heavens I am Still a Woman**   *16*
13. **His Bladder Cancer Disappeared In Front of My Eyes**   *17*
14. **A Chain of Miracles**   *18*
15. **A Choice Between Surgery and Chi-Lel Therapy**   *19*
16. **Just Tell Me, Sir, What Parts of Your Body Were Good?**   *20*
17. **They Used Long Needles to Inject "Brain Juice" Into My Baby's Head**   *21*
18. **You Ought to Be Dead by Now**   *22*
19. **An Attractive Lady With an Unspeakable Secret**   *23*
20. **The Entire City Raised Money for Me**   *24*
21. **Alone, Standing In Deep Snow**   *25*
22. **If It Disappeared By Itself It Couldn't Have Been Cancer**   *26*
23. **The Most Stressful Job in China**   *27*
24. **We Dug Up Our Ancestors' Graves**   *28*
25. **Can You See Through My Body?**   *29*
26. **I Would Rather Die Dancing**   *31*
27. **I Gave Money Away**   *33*
28. **I Was An Old Man at 25 and A Young Man at 52**   *34*
29. **I'll Write to You, But Please Don't Reply**   *35*
30. **I Had Been Waiting Forty Years**   *36*
31. **Please Don't Laugh at Me**   *37*
32. **Let's Face It, You Are Too Old for Anything**   *38*
33. **It Was a Minor Problem**   *39*

34. **Partner, I'll Take Care of You the Next Thirty Years**   *41*
35. **Unexpectedly My Child Stood Up**   *43*
36. **Healing Others, Healing Herself**   *45*
37. **Teased by His Classmate**   *46*
38. **Say Farewell to the Great Wall**   *47*
39. **I Wouldn't Have Been Able Tell Whether You Were a Man Or a Woman**   *49*
40. **An Orange Saved a Professor's Life**   *50*
41. **An Acupuncturist Became a "Barehanded Doctor"**   *51*
42. **I Ate a Lot of Rice**   *52*
43. **I Spat In My Wife's Face**   *53*
44. **A Dead Man's Last Gamble**   *55*
45. **A Skeleton Soldier**   *56*
46. **I Have Only One Bladder, Please Don't Cut It**   *57*
47. **My Wife, Please Don't Let Our Friends Laugh at Us**   *58*
48. **A Young Principal Couldn't Make It to the Bathroom**   *59*
49. **My Aunt Saved Me**   *60*
50. **Welcome Home**   *61*
51. **A Long March**   *62*
52. **Like Floating On Air**   *63*
53. **A Woman Warrior**   *64*
54. **That's My Toe**   *65*
55. **Hey, What's Wrong With You?**   *66*
56. **She Sang After Fifty Years**   *67*
57. **I Had Prepared My Own Funeral Clothes**   *68*
58. **I Don't Want to Leave**   *69*
59. **This Doctor Quit Her Job as a Medicine Dispenser**   *70*
60. **An S-Shaped Creature Transformed Into a Beautiful Girl**   *71*
61. **An Old Martial Arts Champion**   *72*
62. **A Sportsman's Nightmare**   *73*
63. **A New Tooth Grew in an Old Mouth**   *74*
64. **Entering the Back Door to Recovery**   *75*
65. **Sending Chi to Taiwan**   *77*
66. **A Faded Photograph**   *79*
67. **I Spent My Father's Gold Mine**   *81*
68. **Politically Correct**   *82*
69. **A Soldier's Lonely Wife**   *83*
70. **Helping Their Sons Take Examinations**   *85*
71. **The Man Who Likes To Drink Chi**   *87*
72. **Only a Three Day's Supply of Medicine**   *88*
73. **Being Without Money Was a Blessing in Disguise**   *89*
74. **His Pants Dropped In Front of Thousands of People**   *91*
75. **Her Boss Refused to Save Her Life—She's Glad**   *92*
76. **Kidney Stones in a Small Bottle**   *93*
77. **Deja Vu**   *95*

78. Saved By a "Future" Doctor   *96*

79. She Has Inspired 20,000 people   *97*

80. A Predictable Headache   *99*

81. Thrice, My Skull Didn't Crack Like A Nut   *100*

82. Goodbye Wheelchair, Hello Freedom   *101*

83. Misfortune Dropping From the Sky   *103*

84. I Took Chi Instead Of Medicine   *105*

85. Tree of Sweat and Tears   *106*

86. A Japanese Girl Said Good-bye to Her Hearing Aid   *107*

87. Sixth Floor? No Problem!   *108*

88. The Latest Victim of World War   *109*

89. Dear Husband, Please Don't Abandon Me Because I Am Sick   *111*

90. Does My Boyfriend Truly Love Me?   *113*

91. If I Should Die On the Train, So Be It!   *114*

92. More Limber at Sixty Than She Was as a Girl   *115*

93. Born In Hong Kong   *116*

94. A Woman From Inner Mongolia   *117*

95. Taking Care of Daughter, Mother Was Healed   *118*

96. I Feel As If I Were in My Thirties Again   *119*

97. Money Can Buy Surgery But Love Can Heal   *120*

98. An Old Woman Shouldn't Go   *121*

99. Sis, You Married the Right Guy   *122*

100. No More Needles   *123*

101. An Eighty-Year-Old Educator   *124*

Part Two: The Methods

Introduction to the Methods   *126*

1. Lift Chi Up and Pour Chi Down Method   *133*

2. Three Centers Merge Standing Method   *145*

3. Wall Squatting   *149*

4. La Chi   *150*

Pressure Point Diagram   *151*

Chapter One:

The Interviews

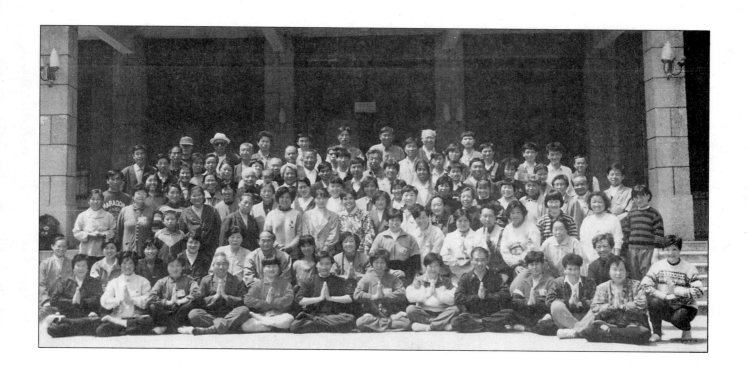

Introduction to the Interviews

When I traveled to the Zhineng Qigong Center in May 1995, I had planned to interview only thirty people. After all, how could one expect to find more than thirty miracles in one place within one month?

Once at the Center, however, with the blessings of Dr. Pang, I was flooded with people who were eager to tell me of their sufferings, struggles and finally triumph over disease. At first I concentrated only on those who had recovered from cancer, but there were so many such examples that I later declined to interview many cancer patients so as to include cases of people with other ailments.

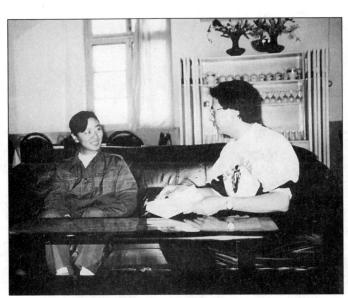

An interview in process

Most of the people I interviewed could name their diseases in exact medical terms because they had spent so much time in conventional hospitals. They knew the technicalities of their illnesses all too well. I long debated with myself over whether I should translate literally all of the Chinese in these accounts into precise English. But finally I realized that the purpose of this book, to inspire others, would be much better served by simply rendering the essence of each story and each person than by striving for some scholarly exactitude. After all, what meaning would each story have without a human face?

I also considered different ways of classifying the stories. First I categorized them by disease, but soon found this difficult because many interviewees had had multiple illnesses. Besides, these stories are more about the triumphs of human beings over affliction than about the diseases which made them suffer. Then I tried to classify the stories according to the duties of the interviewees in the center: teachers, doctors, students (patients), instructor trainees. But these artificial categories lacked meaning. So in the end I decided to present these accounts in more or less the order in which they were written.

There are three things you should know before reading the interviews.

1. Since most of the people I interviewed were healed in the Center, many of these people connect their healings directly to the Center's founder, Lao-shi. This seems only natural, but it would be a mistake to conclude that these people idolize him. As Lao-shi, who is against personal worship, explained during the opening ceremony, "I have only a certain amount of chi, and so do you. If it were my chi alone that could heal, I would be drawn dry. It is the chi which has been gathered here by all of us that heals."

2. Even though most of the miracles in these stories occurred at the Center, I've been told that there have been similar occurrences with Chi-Lel practitioners throughout China. Indeed, spontaneous healings are chi-healing phenomenon which can happen anywhere in the world. Some participants in my workshops in the United States have also experienced instant healing. Yet only a small percentage of people can absorb chi readily enough for an immediate healing. Most people need to work at it, and nothing can replace hard work for "chi helps those who help themselves."

3. Although some of these recoveries are so incredible that they almost amount to resurrections from the dead, Chi Lel is not a panacea that cures everyone.

"Do people die here?" I asked the doctor in charge in the Center. The doctor, now retired from a major hospital, told me that because many people arrive at the Center in the latter stages of disease, some of them do die: "But they die without pain and without being drugged up. Family members are often grateful that their loved ones are able to die in such a dignified way."

I didn't quite comprehend what the doctor was trying to say until one night I accompanied a teacher as he went to emit chi to his students. "How do you feel today?" the teacher asked a middle-aged woman. "I had some bowel movements today, teacher," the student replied, with a hopeful smile. "Good," replied the teacher, emitting chi to her. When it was my turn to emit chi to the student, I accidentally touched her stomach and was stunned to feel that her entire belly was hardened. Later, on our way to our rooms, I asked the teacher what was wrong with the lady.

"She has a spreading stomach cancer. She came here late, and will probably not make it."

"That serious? But I didn't sense any despair in her."

"She is still alive, isn't she? It is a good sign that she is reacting to chi, and I have seen other people cured in similar situations. There is still hope."

Why did the teacher believe that there was still hope for this student? Well, the teacher had been there himself—on the brink of hopelessness. It is this teacher's own recovery which is the subject of the first story of this book.

As you read on, you will find these stories are about suffering, struggle, triumph, courage, friendship, love and hope.

1. If I Live I'll Repay Every Penny I Owe You

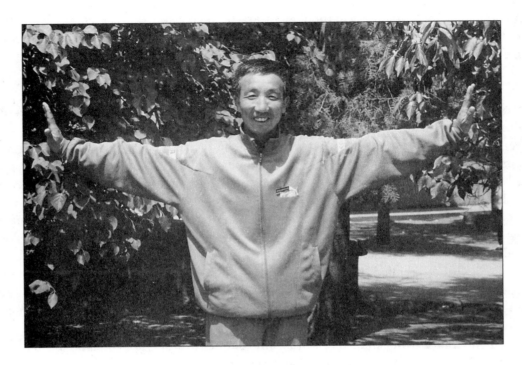

Ren Jing Xiang, 42, teacher

"Are you the one who held his hands up in a straight line at shoulder level for eight and a half hours?" I asked Teacher Ren, for I had heard of his incredible feat. He nodded his head with a smile and instantly we became friends.

"In 1989 I started having heart problems. I didn't dare sleep because as soon as I closed my eyelids my heart stopped. The doctors recommended an angiogram, however, this happened at the time of the June 4th Tiananmen Square incident and the United States had stopped sending much-needed medical supplies. Consequently, I couldn't undergo the angiogram treatment.

"Then in 1991, my heart muscles were damaged further and surgery was recommended. However, the hospital required a deposit of forty-five thousand yuan. Going home to borrow money from friends and relatives, and knowing that my chance of recovery was fair at best, I told everyone 'If I live I'll repay every penny I owe you, but if I die please release my wife of my debt.' It was not until 1993 that I borrowed enough money for the heart surgery. Then on the day of the surgery the doctor in charge advised me that I should wait until the other half of my heart became bad in order that one surgery might take care of the whole heart."

"What do you mean?" I asked Teacher Ren, as he attempted to describe in medical terms the problem with his heart. "Are you telling me that half of your heart, with all of its vessels and valves was bad, and the other half was getting bad too?" He nodded that this was true.

"Did you take the doctor's advice to delay your surgery?"

4

"No, I didn't. I wanted to get it over with because I knew that if I went home without surgery I would end up lying in bed, doing nothing. Such a rich-man's disease I couldn't afford. But my wife insisted that I delay my surgery and go home.

"Although I finally agreed not to have the surgery, I wanted to travel. I had envisioned that someone, somewhere, would cure me. My wife adamantly opposed any traveling, but somehow I got out of the hospital and bought a ticket to the Chi-Lel Center. I had heard of the Center, but only had a vague idea of where it was. On the train I met someone with a broken hand who was also going there. Upon reaching the Center, I witnessed a Chi-Lel teacher ordering this patient to remove his cast and lift a cup! My confidence rose when I saw a broken hand being healed instantly. What else could Chi Lel do?

"Then I settled down in the Center and decided that I would rather die here than vegetate at home. After a few days, I felt very much at home. Then one night, as I was practicing holding my hands up, I told myself that to heal my illness I must have determination. After some time, I felt my heartbeats quieting down. Worried at first, I told myself that I would rather die than put my hands down. As time went on, I felt changes in my heart as its beats and sounds returned to normal. When the cock crowed the next morning, I sensed my heart had completely recovered. I couldn't contain my excitement for a miracle had happened!

"The doctor took an EKG, which confirmed that my heart had indeed returned to normal."

"Teacher Ren, are you telling me that anyone with a severe heart problem can cure themselves by holding their hands up for at least eight and a half hours at one time?"

"All the Chi Lel movements taught here can do the healing."

Was Teacher Ren implying that anyone with faith in Chi Lel can defeat their life-threatening illnesses? I didn't need to ask further, because for him the answer was too obvious.

2. A New Life

Shortly after Ms. Pan graduated from medical college, she was diagnosed with bone cancer in her left leg. She underwent surgery in August 1991 to remove the cancer by "killing the bone"

"Being a young doctor and such an attractive lady, how did you feel when you found out you were ill?"

"At first I couldn't comprehend its ramifications. After all I had the best medical care and a loving family. Yet things went from bad to worse. First, when I woke up from my surgery and looked for my fiancé he was nowhere to be found—he had left during my surgery. But I was strong and wanted to show the world that I was a survivor.

"Following the surgery, I underwent chemotherapy, but after the twelfth treatment, my liver, heart, kidneys, stomach, and almost every internal organ were weakened. Not only my physical body but also my spirit was totally crushed. I was not a living person anymore. It was at this time that someone mentioned Chi Lel. Chi Lel? Previously I would have laughed at such an idea, but now I was ready to try anything. At first I was so weak that someone had to carry me to the Chi-Lel practice, but after the twentieth day I was able to go there by myself. My spirits began to return to me and I felt hope.

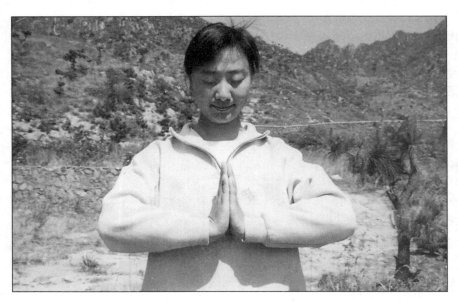

Pan Hung*, M.D.,25, a trainee in the two-year qigong academy

"Then one day I discovered a mysterious swelling on my left shoulder. When it later turned to pus and dissolved, I intuitively knew that my cancer was cured. It was then that I decided to abandon chemotherapy in spite of my family's opposition. After a few months practice, I had completely recovered—not only was I cancer free but also my supposedly dead bone somehow reestablished itself with nerve fibers and blood vessels, and became alive again. It is truly a miracle.

"Because my case is well known in my hometown, local officials have decided to introduce Chi Lel to all levels of this municipality's government and schools."

"Why did you come to study at this academy?"

"A friend came here first and then asked me to come."

Later I found out that her friend was an assistant Chi-Lel teacher who had met Dr. Pan while she was terribly ill. He had encouraged her and nourished her back to health. Naturally, love had developed between these two young people.

"What would you like to do after graduation?"

"I want to devote the rest of my life to Chi Lel."

Deep in my heart, I have no doubt of her sincerity.

* Dr. Pan demonstrates the Chi-Lel methods in Part Two of this book.

3. What Miracle Drug from the West Have You Taken?

Upon first meeting Teacher Liu, I was impressed with her total dedication to her work as a Chi-Lel teacher.

"Teacher Liu, being so young, pretty and smart, you certainly could accomplish a lot in the outside world. Why, therefore, are you so earnest about serving the sick?"

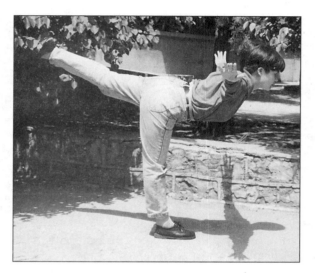

Liu Xiao-Jun*, 23, teacher

"Without Chi Lel, my mother would have died." She was referring to her mother, Young Chi-Min, 48, a school teacher. "Back in June 1990, my mother was diagnosed with breast cancer. Upon hearing the news, my whole family except for my mother, who pretended to be strong, cried from despair. Later, after she had already undergone surgery twice, her cancer reappeared even while she was still in the hospital. The doctors then predicted she had only two or three years to live.

"Then one of our friends told us that Lao-shi was coming to town to give a lecture on Chi Lel. We didn't believe in Chi Lel and dismissed the idea of going. Yet one of my mother's students persisted, urging us that we had nothing to lose. So we went. After the lecture, Lao-shi asked the audience, 'Have you touched your tumors to see if they have softened, become smaller or disappeared?'

"I saw tears coming from my mother's eyes as she touched her left breast. The lump was gone! We embraced each other and cried with joy. In fact, my mother hadn't told us that her cancer had already spread to her left breast.

"When my mother returned to the hospital for a checkup, the doctor was shocked to find no trace of cancer. The doctor asked, 'Teacher Young, what miracle drug from the West have you taken?' When my mother told him the truth, the doctor didn't believe her. But no matter, my mother is still alive after five years."

Besides showing great care towards her patients, Ms. Liu is also an avid learner. She is currently studying English in order to be able to help the sick, from wherever they may come.

Teacher Liu and her mother

*Teacher Liu demonstrates La Chi in Part Two of this book.

4. I Want to Live—I Have Three Young Children at Home.

"I am a traditional Chinese doctor. In my mid-thirties, I developed severe headaches, stomachaches, and breathing and vision problems. In addition, I developed an irregular heartbeat and worst of all, was diagnosed with breast cancer in 1982. Two years later both my breasts were swelling with painful tumors. Being a doctor, I undertook all kinds of treatments but without success. In the end I simply remained helplessly at home."

"Was your family supportive?"

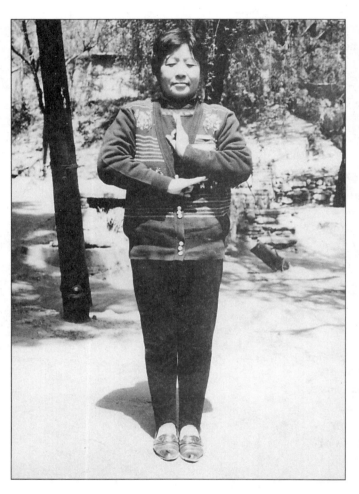

Liang Gui-Zhi, M.D., 49, teacher

After hearing my question, Dr. Liang sobbed and replied, "No, my mother-in-law wrote me off as dead and encouraged my husband to find another woman. I prayed to different gods to let me live for the sake of my three young children—I even prayed to Chairman Mao!"

"How did you find Chi Lel?"

"After my mother-in-law and husband treated me so badly, I began to lose hope. I was longing for love and human sympathy. Then one day a neighbor, a Chi-Lel teacher, asked me if I believed in Chi Lel. Even though I didn't know what Chi Lel was, I nodded my head, happy to have finally met someone who seemed genuinely caring. She emitted chi to me and instantly I felt better. Finding myself smiling, I thought I'd gone crazy! But I had finally found some measure of inner joy and hope after so many years of suffering. And so it was, during January of 1985, that I decided to learn Chi Lel in spite of my family's objections. The next few years, I practiced Chi Lel diligently and gradually regained my health. For the past two years, I have been without any trace of cancer."

"What's happened between you and your husband?"

"We are still married and my husband is happy that we have both regained our black hair."

Dr. Liang also told me that last winter she taught Chi Lel to hundreds of people in her hometown and donated all the proceeds to the Center. In fact, the amount of money she donated was more than her entire yearly salary. Why did she do that? "Chi Lel saved my life, I can never fully repay such a debt."

5. Being Deaf Is a Horrible Thing

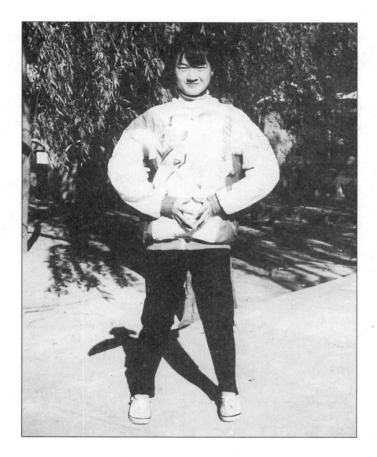

Chen Ming, 14, student

As I interviewed this active, talkative girl, I could hardly believe that she had been a withdrawn child just one month ago. Her dramatic transformation came about when she regained her hearing.

"When I was two years old I had a high fever. The medicine the doctor gave me to cure my fever also caused me to lose my hearing. Even though I sat in the front row at school, I could hardly hear the teachers speak. In addition, I heard noises all the time, which bothered me very much. Naturally, I couldn't keep up with the other classmates. Although my mother took me to several different hospitals, none could heal me.

"Then someone told my mother about the Center and she immediately brought me here. My hearing started improving the first day I arrived here. I practice my Chi-Lel routine daily, never missing a session, and now hear normally without any noises in my ears."

"How did your mother react when she learned that you could hear?"

"She cried and told me that I would get a decent husband after all." Ms. Chen smiled shyly and added, "Believe me, being deaf is a horrible thing."

Of course I believed her. Moreover, I knew that recovering her hearing must have been a joyful and precious experience.

6. I Would Do Anything If Only I Could Stay Here

Ms. Hu went into shock when her husband was killed in a coal mining accident in 1988. After that her health took a dive. She developed low blood pressure, anemia, stomachaches, and back pain. She couldn't raise her head because of a bone spur on one of her neck vertebrae.

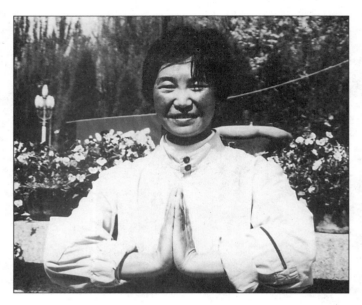

Hu Yun-Ying, 37, housekeeper

"Three years later, just when I thought time was healing my wounds, another tragedy struck. This time I lost my mind. I was deeply depressed and needed someone to look after me around the clock."

"What happened, Ms. Hu?"

She looked down on the ground, said in a choking voice, "My son died."

A year later, my brother heard of the Center and brought me here. At first I cried each time my teacher asked me to relax and I couldn't remember the Chi-Lel movements because as soon as I learned them I forgot them immediately. But my teacher was very patient and supportive. Slowly I began to trust the people around me, and I also started to remember the movements.

"Even though I was much better after two months of Chi Lel, I was still afraid to be left alone. Then one day during one of

Lao-shi's speeches, I saw Lao-shi wave his hand in a sweeping motion. I suddenly felt as if his hand had gone through my head and my mind became instantly clear. A smile came to my face and I told my brother that he could go home now.

"After the third month, I was free to go. Yet I didn't want to leave and implored my teacher, 'I would do anything to stay here.' He replied that the Center was looking for a good housekeeper. 'I'll take the job!' I shouted with joy.

"When I went home for a visit, my relatives were surprised to see me alone, asking, 'How could you have come home by yourself?' They still regarded me as a confused soul!"

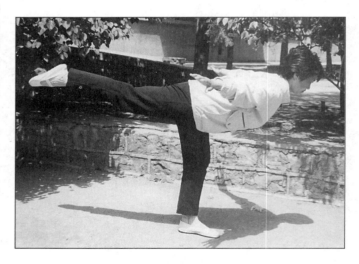

Ms. Hu shows her balance

Like many others at the Center, Ms. Hu serves silently, contributing whatever she can to make this place a comfortable home for the weary and sick.

7. The Taming of the Shrew

When I saw Teacher Liu gracefully leading her folkdancing class, I could hardly believe that she was once paralyzed from the waist down.

"In 1982, I was hit by a car and suffered multiple body injuries. I underwent several operations and spent several months in a hospital convalescing. As soon as I was released from the hospital, I developed arthritis. After that, my body was in constant pain and my blood circulation was so inadequate that I wore insulated shoes on hot days just to keep my feet warm.

"I'd always had a bad temper, even before the car accident. In fact, I was known for hitting my mother-in-law with my fists. So, at age thirty-seven, I was one angry woman, always ready to pounce on people with little or no provocation.

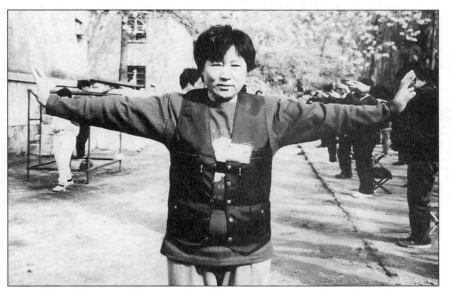

Liu Ji-Hung, 50, teacher

"A few years later, just when I thought I had suffered enough, my body suddenly became paralyzed from the waist down. Unable even to turn-over, I lay in a hospital bed, staring at the ceiling day and night as pain kept me awake. After being in the hospital for two months without improvement, I began to have the horrible thought that I would spend the rest of life just as I was.

"Then a visitor of my hospital roommate took pity on me and showed me the La Chi (opening and closing hands) movement. Since my hands had limited movement, I mainly used my imagination to carry out the motions. I visualized the blue sky when opening and the inside of my body when closing. After spending hours imagining these maneuvers, I found I could fall into a normal sleep. With such encouragement, I began to practice the movements whenever I was awake.

"On the ninth day of practice, my left leg suddenly made a jerking motion! It shocked me and I bowed many times to heaven because I thought some divine beings had intervened.

"I continued to practice the movement and, three days later, I could sit up. A week later, I was out of the hospital and had joined our local Chi-Lel group. Within two years, all my ailments were gone. I have been teaching classes since 1991."

"Now that your strength has returned, I would be afraid if I were your mother-in-law," I asked jokingly.

Teacher Liu replied, "I'm not a shrew anymore. My mother-in-law and I are good friends now and we do a lot of things together. Indeed, good moral character is a prerequisite for being a good Chi-Lel practitioner. Occasionally, when I raise my voice at home, my husband immediately reminds me, 'Remember Lao-shi's teachings on the virtue of controlling our temper.' This works every time because whenever Lao-shi's name is mentioned, I become deeply emotional. Without Lao-shi, my life would be a waste."

Indeed, Chi Lel had not only helped Teacher Liu physically but also morally.

8. An Ultrasound Specialist

I first encountered Dr. Wang when she was monitoring an ultrasound machine while three Chi-Lel teachers were treating patients. After all the others had gone, Dr. Wang began to tell me her story.

"In my hometown, I was an ultrasound machine specialist in a major hospital. When I retired from work a year ago, Lao-shi asked me to come to the Center. Without hesitation, I agreed. I also persuaded my husband, an internist and an X-ray specialist, to come with me."

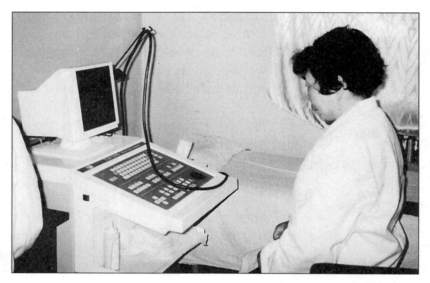

Wang Feng-Yun, M.D., 61

"Why were you so enthusiastic about coming to the Center?"

"I believe that Chi Lel is an excellent way of treating many chronic illnesses. I had arthritis, severe back pain and many other illnesses before I practiced Chi Lel. As I was working in a hospital, I could obtain the most advanced medicine from all over the world but all these medicines were powerless in treating my illnesses. I relied so much on drugs that I sometimes wondered whether it was I or my medicines that were in charge of my body. As a doctor, I also know that the side effects of some of these drugs were very harmful.

"So I was looking for an alternative way of healing myself. When a former patient came to see me, I could hardly believe what I saw. My previously spiritless patient had been transformed into a healthy, energetic person. He talked about Chi Lel as if it were a panacea for all ailments. So I decided to come to the Center to experience it for myself. Once in the Center, I forgot that I was a doctor and worked just as hard as anybody else fighting my diseases. Abandoning my belief that plenty of rest was good for the sick, I would practice Chi Lel until I was sweating profusely; the more pain I felt the more I practiced. After a few months, I was completely cured. I am grateful to Chi Lel."

"So have you abandoned traditional medicine?"

"No, I think both Chi Lel and modern medicine have their own merits. They will come together at some point in the future. In fact, they have already done so, as you witnessed today, when I monitored the ultrasound machine while Chi-Lel teachers were treating patients.

"What do doctors do here?"

"We attend to emergency cases, but the core of our job is to diagnose patients when they first come in and again when they finish their twenty-four days of training. In this hospital, we doctors are playing a supporting role because the patients are actively involved in their own healing process. Since no drugs are prescribed, there are no jobs for pharmacists either."

"How about diet? Are there any special eating habits or special food for different patients?"

"No, there aren't any special diets or foods requirements. Students can eat whatever they please. Of course, they know what to avoid for their special illnesses."

At the Center, there are no medicines or special diets, just sweat, love, and plenty of chi.

9. Military Man Ordered Daughter to Go

Ms. Huang, being the only daughter of a military family, was trained to have strict discipline and self-control. When she discovered herself becoming languid at school she dismissed it as laziness. But as her condition worsened, her father took her to a hospital for a checkup—it was leukemia.

"I wasn't afraid of the ailment because I was young and otherwise healthy. The doctors recommended chemotherapy and I was glad to comply. During the four-month treatment, my illness was brought under control. But it reappeared as soon as the treatment was stopped. We lost confidence in Western medicine and tried Chinese herbal medicine. That didn't work either and my illness became worse. We returned to the Western doctors and they suggested that I have a bone marrow transplant."

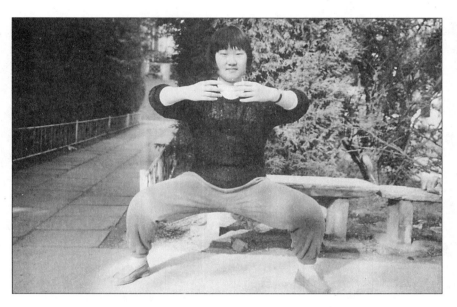

Huang Xiao-Yun, 18, instructor trainee

"Did you go through with the operation?"

"No, they didn't have the right type of bone marrow. Besides, there was no way for us to come up with the 150,000 yuan required for the treatment."

"So you turned to Chi Lel out of necessity?"

"No, in fact, I was opposed to Chi Lel. I thought it was superstitious and only good for the old. When my father mentioned Chi Lel to me I felt rebellious. I was very surprised when my father became enthusiastic about Chi Lel after talking about it with a friend of his. He used to think like me—had he lost his mind? I wondered.

"But nothing could change my father's military mind once it was made up. So I was forced to go to the Center in August 1994. However, while I was on the train to the Center, my attitude changed. I thought it might be a good thing to see more of the world before I died. Besides, I wanted my father to have good memories of me, not to think of me as a disobedient child.

"After I arrived at the Center, I met many people who had been miraculously healed. My eyes opened and I began to believe. I realized that, after all, Chi Lel is not only for the old but for me too.

"Once I found my purpose here, I practiced Chi Lel assiduously. After two months of Chi-Lel therapy, my leukemia went into remission; after two more months, I became cancer free. Now I am completing a three-month instructor's training course. After that I want to enter the two-year program at the Chi-Lel Academy. I have bonded to this place and I don't want to leave."

10. I Have Returned

When Ms. Ma was diagnosed with breast cancer, she followed the standard hospital treatment: surgery, chemotherapy, and radiation. Unfortunately, this treatment did not stop the spread of cancer to her bones.

"My cancer was out of control and I was in a desperate situation. When someone told me about the Chi-Lel Center, I immediately took a train here. I expected it to be similar to a regular hospital with the Chi-Lel masters taking care of me while I spent most of my time in bed. However, I was somewhat disappointed to find that the prescription for my illness was hard work."

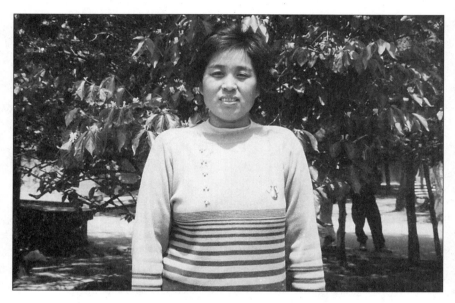

Ma Chiao, 42, student

"Weren't you impressed with the testimonies of people who had achieved extraordinary benefits from working hard on Chi Lel?"

"Yes, this gave me hope and courage to follow the daily routine. But my hope dimmed when I found I wasn't improving that much compared with my classmates. I began to question why I should work myself into exhaustion every day instead of resting comfortably at home. So after staying at the Center for one month, I went home.

"For the first few days at home, I was glad that I was getting plenty of rest. However, I soon realized getting out of bed was becoming more and more difficult as my illness progressed. In the Center, I was able to put in eight hours of Chi Lel fighting my disease; at home, I could hardly go down the stairs without feeling fatigued.

"Realizing that I was only vegetating to death at home, I returned to the Center with a new appreciation of its value. Where before I had acted as an unwilling participant, now I became an active member of the group. I worked diligently every day, helping my classmates whenever possible, and feeling happy when another's illness disappeared instead of jealous. Indeed, helping others with their illnesses made mine seem manageable. No longer did I regard practices such as singing songs and marching like an army as brainwashing. In fact, everything done in the Center seemed designed to help me as an individual to recover. With a changed attitude, I began to notice the symptoms of my cancer disappearing. I now understood that recovery has a lot to do with willingness to help oneself and others."

"So no pain no gain? Ms. Ma?"

"That's right. And I want to add: No love no gain."

11. Double Happiness

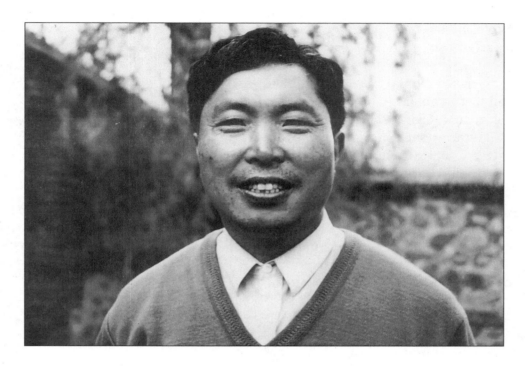

Zhao An, 42, student

"In 1988, I became very weak, and my stomach expanded with frequent vomiting and loss of appetite. I was diagnosed with sclerosis of the liver. During the next two years I was in and out of the hospital, spending more than 35,000 yuan. Although I was still weak, my illness was brought under control in 1991.

"Unfortunately, my illness reappeared last September. I was scared because I couldn't afford another prolonged stay in the hospital. Just when I had nowhere to turn I encountered an old hospital roommate. 'You look so young and healthy. Where have you been?' I asked. He told me that he had learned Chi Lel in the Center and that his liver had already been healed for several years.

"Chi Lel? I thought that was only good for old folks who had nothing to do. But seeing my friend's amazing transformation, I eagerly wanted to try Chi Lel too. Immediately, my wife and I, along with my sister-in-law, took a train to the Center.

"In less than a month, my appetite returned and I felt very happy. The doctors tell me that my liver is now functioning normally. Not only was my liver saved, but also my sister-in-law's ovarian tumor disappeared (see next interview). It was truly a double happiness."

12. Thank Heaven I Am Still a Woman

Ms. Jia told me that her left ovary had been surgically removed six years ago because of a tumor.

"The tumor weighed more than ten pounds, and was so painful that I couldn't move. When it was removed I was greatly relieved, and believed that I would never suffer from such an ailment again.

"Unfortunately, a short time later another tumor appeared in my right ovary. It was growing fast and the doctors suggested that the ovary be removed. I was horrified because without ovaries, I would become a man.

"Then my sister and brother-in-law (previous interview) told me that they were going to learn Chi Lel at the Center and asked me to come with them. I agreed because my brother-in-law is the brains of the family and whatever he does makes sense to me.

"Before I arrived at the Center, the size of my tumor was 6x7 cm. After a few days of practicing Chi Lel, I felt great pain in my ovary, but then the pain disappeared. When a doctor later did an ultrasound on me, she couldn't find any trace of the tumor inside my ovary.

"Thank heaven I am still a woman!"

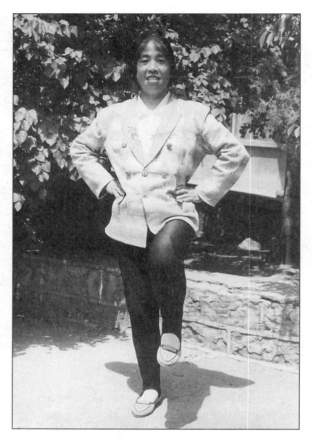

Jia Ching-Zhi, 42, student

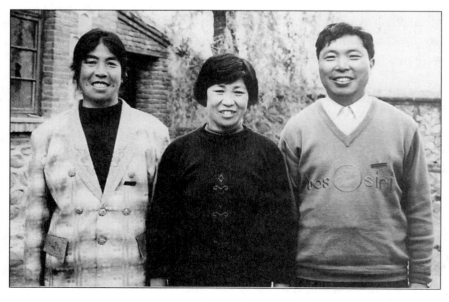

Jia Ching-Zhi with sister and brother-in-law

16

13. His Bladder Cancer Disappeared In Front of My Eyes

When Mr. Wen was diagnosed with a malignant tumor in his bladder, doctors suggested surgery to remove the tumor, followed by chemotherapy and radiation treatment.

"But when the doctors told me that not even surgery was a guarantee for a cancer-free future, I began looking for an alternative treatment.

"Luckily, a friend told me about Chi Lel. Immediately, in March, I took a two-day train trip to the Center, determined that I would rather die in the Center than waste away with cancer at home. But after the first month of training, I was dismayed when doctors told me that the size of my tumor had actually increased, rather than decreased as I had hoped."

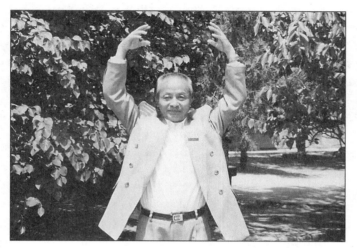

Wen Guang-Li, 57, student

"Were you discouraged?"

"Not discouraged, but puzzled. I had been practicing Chi Lel diligently with a 100 percent effort. What was wrong? After discussing it with my teacher, I realized that illnesses react to chi in different ways, sometimes becoming worse before they get better.

"In addition to encouraging me to continue practicing Chi Lel, my teacher also advised me to visualize blue sky instead of focusing on my illness while practicing. So I followed my teacher's instruction, forgetting my illness. When the second month's report came, I was happy to find my tumor down to half its original size.

"Then on the ninth of this month, my teacher asked me if I wanted to have chi treatment by four teachers simultaneously while being monitored on-line with an ultrasound machine. I jumped at the chance. They also told me of an American friend who would be videotaping the procedure. I guess the American friend must have been you since you were videotaping while I was being treated."

Indeed, I was fortunate to witness the world's foremost on-line surgery using chi. Using an ultrasound machine, doctors put Mr. Wen's bladder cancer on a TV monitor and four teachers began to emit chi. Within a few seconds, the cancer began to shrink. In less than a minute, Mr. Wen's bladder cancer literally disappeared in front of my eyes! I was stunned and couldn't immediately comprehend what was going on. That morning, they treated eight students with tumors. Of those, five disappeared and one became smaller while two were unaffected. A doctor told me that it was their best record so far.

Was the ultrasound machine working normally? Were the tumors only disappearing temporarily? I took the view of a skeptic and asked the doctor if he would look at these tumors again ten days later in my presence. Using the ultrasound machine a second time, the doctor couldn't find any trace of those tumors which had been successfully removed using chi.

Who knows what the future holds for this way of treating malignant and non-malignant tumors? Just like any progressive hospital in the world, the Center is conducting ongoing clinical research. One thing is sure: with thousands of students being treated daily, the Center will find better ways to treat diseases using Chi-Lel therapy. Indeed, it has been silently leading the world in new ways of treating many chronic diseases. Now it is up to the world to catch up with what's going on there.

After Mr. Wen finished his treatment, I asked how he felt at the time. "I didn't feel pain or any other special sensation. I just felt happy."

14. A Chain of Miracles

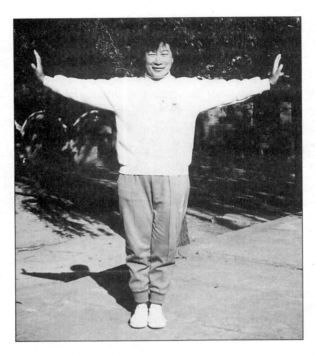

Lin Shua-Hua, 54, teacher

In 1972, Teacher Lin underwent surgery to remove a benign tumor in her throat. The tumor reappeared five years later, spreading to her esophagus. It was so painful that she couldn't eat solid food. In 1983, she underwent further surgery and lost her voice. Seven years later, the tumor reappeared and this time it was malignant, and she became immobilized and had to be fed intravenously. Eventually she weighed only seventy-nine pounds, a mere skeleton.

"When the doctors told my husband that there was nothing more they could do for me, I gave up all hope of survival. I merely laid in bed, in terrible pain, waiting to die.

"So when my son suggested that I learn Chi Lel I was in no mood to listen. However, my son was so persistent that I finally agreed to try it. At first I needed three people to carry me to Chi-Lel practice, but after twenty days I was able to go there by myself. When my stomach began to hurt a lot my teacher reassured me that it was a good development, and that I was responding to chi. Incredibly, within three months I had regained my health! When I went back to my doctors for a checkup they couldn't believe their eyes, for I had survived against all odds."

"Why was your son so persistent in persuading you to learn Chi Lel?"

"Because he himself had been cured of a strange illness. He used to wear gloves to school because his hands had many tiny flesh particles hanging from them. But after practicing Chi Lel for fifteen days, his hands were cured."

"In addition, my son told me that our Chi-Lel teacher had also been saved by Chi Lel. In 1986 when Lao-shi came to our city, three quarters of her heart was not functioning and her skin was almost black. After listening to Lao-shi, she began to study Chi Lel and recovered completely."

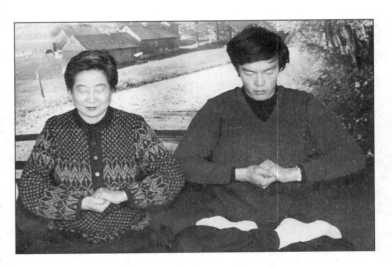

Teacher Lin's son and their teacher

Indeed, as I was to encounter again and again at the Center, a chain of miracles had occurred.

15. A Choice Between Surgery and Chi-Lel Therapy

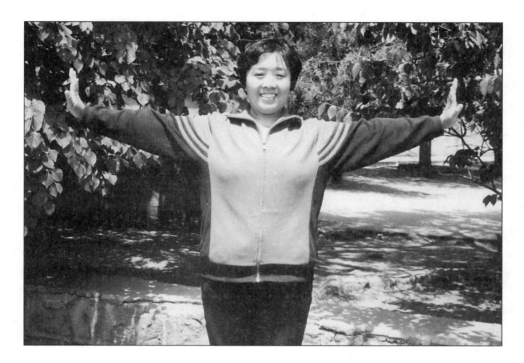

Zhang Li-En, 42, student

When Ms. Zhang was diagnosed with breast cancer, for her sister, a medical doctor, the choice was obvious: remove the cancer immediately. So naturally, when Ms. Zhang told her sister that she was considering Chi-Lel therapy, her sister replied, "Are you crazy? This is life and death. If you wait, the cancer will surely spread to other areas, and then it will be too late to save your life. It's not that I'm against Chi Lel, but you need to do the sure thing."

In contrast, Ms. Zhang's husband was a staunch Chi-Lel practitioner. He advised her, "Surgery cannot guarantee that the cancer won't reappear. If Chi Lel doesn't cure you, it will at least suppress the cancer."

"So your sister advised you to do the 'sure' thing while your husband urged you act on faith?"

"Yes, and I chose Chi Lel."

"Why?"

"I believe in Chi Lel. Although I had been doing some Chi Lel since 1990, during the last two years I had neglected my practice. Nevertheless, I believed that with persistent work I could heal myself. So upon coming to the Center two months ago, I practiced Chi Lel from very early in the morning to very late at night, determined to defeat my cancer.

"When I went back to my doctors for an extensive checkup they couldn't find any trace of cancer. I have been pronounced cancer free and my sister is very happy for me."

"Besides studying hard, what other techniques do you use?"

"While doing the Chi-Lel movements I imagine that all my pressure points are enlarged into big tunnels which allow chi to pass in and out easily. Try it, it works."

16. Just Tell Me, Sir, What Parts of Your Body Were Good?

Mr. Shen was a very friendly old man. It was hard to imagine that only a year ago this healthy gentleman was little better than dead.

"Since 1959, I have had many surgeries," Mr. Shen began, showing me his scars. "The nerves

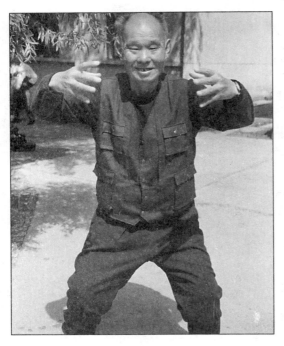

in my head above the ears hurt so much that it took two surgeries to calm them. Every night for the last twenty years, I needed sleeping pills to sleep. Many of my neck and back vertebrae were either dislocated or had bone spurs. It was very painful and I couldn't move my hands freely. I had heart problems; my stomach and intestines were bad; and I had gallstones."

As Mr. Shen talked on, I laughed and said jokingly, "Just tell me, sir, what parts of your body were good?"

Mr. Shen, who didn't know I was joking, replied, "Only my liver and pancreas." He then laughed and began to tell me how he had conquered his illnesses.

"One day I accidentally stumbled upon Lao-shi's book on Chi Lel, and immediately was sold on the idea that Chi Lel could heal me. So during the next five months, I spent every waking minute of my life practicing Chi Lel. Gradually my illnesses, one after another, succumbed to the power of chi. Now I sleep well and feel thirty years younger."

"What are you doing here in the Center?"

"I am taking the three-month training on how to use chi to help others. In fact, I healed a baby with paralysis

Shen Shi-Rong, 74, instructor trainee

the other day."

When I showed him the name of a child I had interviewed the other day, he said excitedly,"That's him! That's him!" (see next interview).

"Would you emit chi to me as you did to the child?" I requested. Mr. Shen gladly complied, and I felt his chi turning circles inside my head. I thanked him sincerely. Perhaps someday I will be able to use this same technique to cure a paralyzed child.

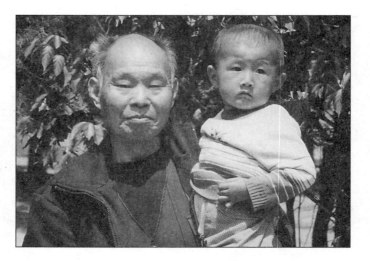

Mr. Shen holds the child he healed

17. They Used Long Needles to Inject "Brain Juice" Into My Baby's Head

A child was running everywhere, waiting for his turn to be interviewed. It was hard to believe that just two weeks ago this baby could barely move. His mother told me that three of her son's fingers had been crooked, his legs were bent into an X-shape, and, because he lacked an appetite, his growth had been stagnant.

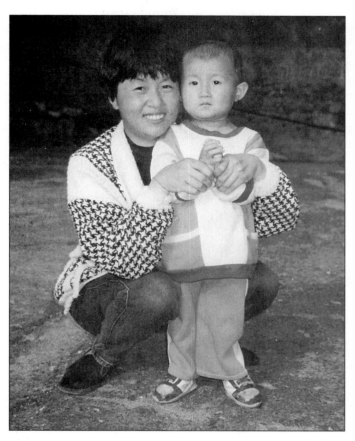

Tian Li-Bao with his mother

"I cried each time I saw doctors using long needles to inject 'brain juice' into my baby's head. They told me that the lower part of my son's brain had somehow moved to the left, pressing some nerves and resulting in partial body paralysis.

"But the medicine had no effect on my child at all. My husband and I didn't know what to do. We couldn't have another child because of the government's one-child policy. So we turned to Chi Lel."

"How did you find out about the Chi-Lel Center?"

"One of my relatives in Beijing is a Chi-Lel practitioner and he emitted chi to my child. My son responded well; he was able to turn his body after receiving the chi. So I decided to bring him here for further chi therapy. A few days ago my son was able to walk freely after receiving chi from someone. He eats a lot now and I am very happy."

"Does your son believe in chi?"

"How could he? He is less than two years old."

"So chi also works on nonbelievers?"

"I don't know. As long as I believe in Chi Lel, my son will get the benefits."

When the child grows up, I wonder whether he will believe what happened to him?

18. You Ought to Be Dead by Now

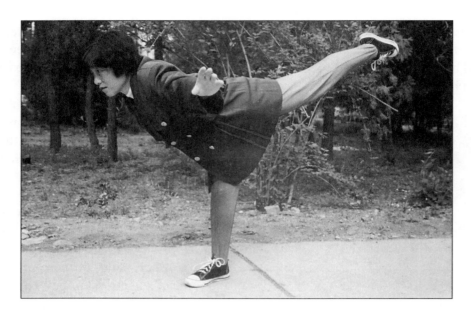

Liu Zhao-Ying, 38, instructor trainee

When Ms. Liu told me the name of the major illness she had, I didn't recognize it. Even when she wrote the name down, I still didn't get it. "Well, put it this way, it is as serious as having an incurable cancer. Three of us in our village had this disease at the same time; two died a long time ago and I am the only survivor." That got my attention.

"In 1985, I developed arthritis along with this disease (later I learned she had systemic lupus), and my health went downhill. My digestive, vascular, nervous, and nearly every other system of my body went bad. I felt pain if someone touched one of my muscles; my hands looked as if I were dead; I wore winter clothes in the summertime.

"A hospital became my regular home. Daily I saw dead bodies being carried away from this horrible place. When would it be my turn? I was afraid of death—who doesn't want to live?

"One day a relative of my hospital roommate suggested that Chi Lel could bring hope to me. So, accompanied by my little brother, I came to the Center in March 1993. After two months of Chi-Lel therapy, I could take care of myself and my brother went home. After a few more months, I had completely recovered. When I returned to my village, many people came to see the miracle of my recovery and asked me to teach them Chi Lel. Instantly I became a famous teacher in my village, and many sick people were healed by doing Chi Lel diligently. They believed in the curative effect of Chi Lel because they had witnessed my transformation.

"When I went back to my doctor in the hospital, he was very surprised to find me still alive, asking, 'Is that you, Ms. Liu? You ought to be dead by now.'"

"Did you tell him to inform his patients with similar illnesses that there is an alternative way of getting out of their death traps?"

"He should do so without me telling him."

I wonder if the doctor will be inclined to do anything—What do you think?

19. An Attractive Lady With an Unspeakable Secret

"I kept my secret for more than ten years, but when my boyfriend proposed to me, I warned him: 'Before you decide to marry me, I have a secret to tell you.' My boyfriend, prepared for the worst, laughed when I whispered, 'I wet the bed at night.' We were married a few months later."

"So you'd been wetting the bed all your life?"

"No, it started when I was thirteen. My mother thought I was just too lazy to get up at night and would beat me. At first I was afraid to go to sleep at night, but as my infirmity continued, my family eventually got used to it. Because I was shy, I never saw a doctor.

"My situation got worse as I grew older. I was afraid to drink water because a glass of water meant many trips to the restroom, up to twenty-one times. It seemed to me that more water came out of my body than what I took in; my lips were often crispy from dehydration. My husband was very supportive and he always made sure that I drank at least some water. We had a son two years after we married and that was when I began to see a doctor.

"Western doctors could offer nothing except the possibility of surgery. Yet they also told me that surgery might not work because I was too old and that the success rate of this surgery wasn't that encouraging. So I turned to acupuncture. The acupuncturists put long needles in many tender places in my body including my toes and back. I underwent this uncomfortable treatment for a few months, but it didn't help. Now I shrink even at the thought of needles.

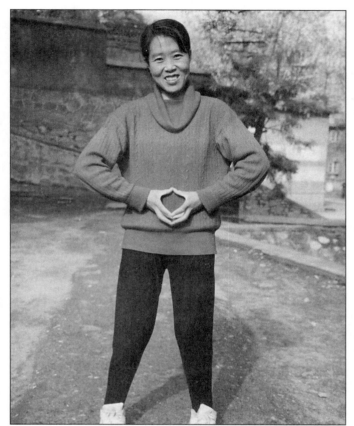

Fan Xu-Mei, 33, student

"What hurt me more was that my son, eight years old, began to carry my burden. When I overheard someone asking who had wet the bed and my son answering that he had done it, I cried. It made me more determined than ever to find a cure. Then a colleague told me about someone with cancer who had been cured at the Center. So I came here at the beginning of this month to give it a try.

"With high hopes, I expected to be cured after shaking hands with Lao-shi, but I wet my bed that night as usual. I was greatly disappointed and told my teacher how I felt. He replied, 'You have just started Chi Lel and yet you expect to be healed at once?'

"So I calmed down and began my Chi-Lel training in earnest. I needed only three hours of sleep every night and the rest of the time I was doing Chi Lel. Now I feel as if I am walking on chi and my whole body is very light. I haven't wet my bed for some time now and I've started drinking water like everybody else, without frequent trips to the restroom. I can lead a normal life now."

In bondage to the restroom for twenty years, Ms. Fan was free at last!

20. The Entire City Raised Money for Me

Ms. Li was an ideal daughter—kind, considerate, good at sports, and an excellent student. But like lightning, leukemia struck her suddenly one day in 1994 during her summer holiday. She was in her third year at college. Even though the doctors recommended chemotherapy they explained that her chances of being cured were minimal because 82 percent of her cells were bad. Nevertheless, she underwent three months of chemotherapy. Her condition did not improve.

"I was lying like a vegetable in a hospital bed—it was very disheartening. The doctors recommended a bone marrow transplant, but my family couldn't afford it.

"When my college classmates found out about my plight, each of them donated fifty yuan to my surgery fund; when the dean of our college became aware of my case, he asked the entire college to help me; when the mayor of our city heard of my situation, he organized a fund raising campaign for me." Ms. Li broke down at this point, saying softly, "They all loved me."

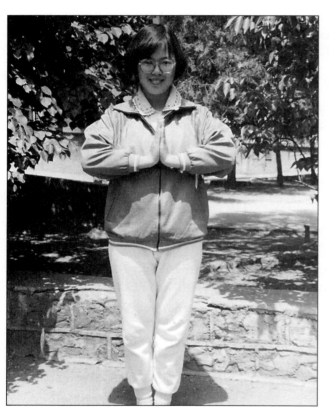

Li Ji-Hung, 22, student

"How did you come to the Center?"

"When I returned to my school to say thank you for their generous support, one of my classmates told me about Chi Lel. I then made up my mind that I would try Chi Lel. However, my family argued with me bitterly. They wanted me to undergo the operation even though the doctor had told them that the chance of any successful recovery was less than 50 percent. Besides it would cost more than 120,000 yuan, not to mention considerable pain and agony. I told my parents that it was my life I was gambling. Still they didn't give in. So I told them that if Chi Lel didn't work I would listen to them.

"I started Chi Lel in November of 1994. One month later, Lao-shi came to teach in our city and I had a chance to shake hands with him. After shaking his hand, I had seven or eight bowel movements in a row. Yet the more I went to the bathroom the happier I became because I knew chi was working on me.

"Last month I came to the Center for more vigorous Chi-Lel training. Now the doctors tell me that my cells are normal. What a relief!"

"Do you have a special way of thinking while doing Chi Lel?"

"Before and after each Chi-Lel routine, I always tell myself that I am fine and imagine that Lao-shi is nearby. When I do the closing movements, I think of my bone marrow. When I do the opening, I think of myself disappearing into the universe."

Ms. Li also told me that twenty-six out of forty of her college classmates took up Chi Lel upon hearing of her miraculous recovery. I wonder how many people in her city who have been inspired by her story will eventually experience miracles themselves.

21. Alone, Standing In Deep Snow

When Teacher Li told me of the ailments she once had, I couldn't keep up with her Chinese. So I asked her to write them down in my notebook and she produced a long list of serious illnesses.

"I was born with an incomplete heart muscle, and had a heart attack at the early age of thirteen. Though my ailing heart was my main problem, I also had arthritis, stomachaches, backaches, depression, pain in my spleen, and a year-round low fever.

"In 1982, my liver shrank and I was hospitalized for five months. My family spent New Year's day with me in the hospital. I had three near-death emergencies that year. With my weight down to only eighty-five pounds, I couldn't even lift a kitchen knife. I became a vegetable at home, without any hope of getting better. Not wanting to burden my family, I thought of suicide. But I was so weak that I couldn't even kill myself, and so chose to die by silently refusing to eat.

"My husband saw through my intention and tried very hard to feed me. But I refused, pretending to be unable to take food. Then one morning my two sons, six and eleven, approached me, one carrying a bowl of milk and a spoon, the other holding a towel. While one tried to feed me the other wiped up spills. With tears in my eyes, I touched my sons and swore silently that I would not let them grow up motherless.

"So my will to live returned to me. One day I discovered many people practicing Chi Lel in a park. I joined the group and plunged into Chi-Lel practice right away. Neither rain nor snow could stop me from coming to class. I remember one morning during a severe snowstorm, I was the only one who showed up for the class. Undaunted, I closed my eyes and began my exercise as usual. At the end, when I opened my eyes, I found myself standing there alone in the park, my feet covered with snow.

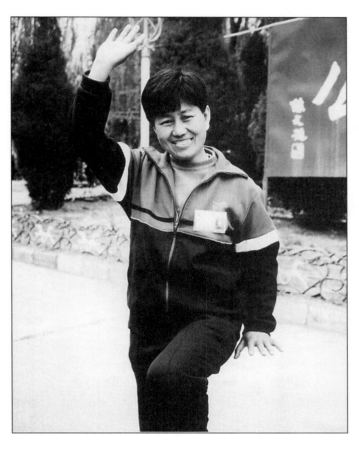

Li Ai-Xiang, 48, teacher

"With Chi-Lel practice, I gradually regained my health. I came to the Center in 1987 for three months of training, and since then have never looked back. I became a teacher three years ago and am now a normal person."

Ms. Li may be a normal person, but she has had an extraordinary experience.

22. If It Disappeared By Itself It Couldn't Have Been Cancer

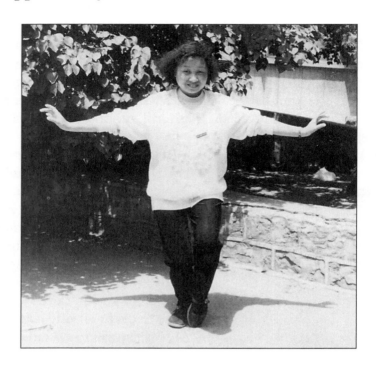

Wu Zhong-Chiong, 43, teacher

"Four years ago I was diagnosed with breast cancer and told that I had only three months to live. I cried and couldn't eat for three days."

"Did your doctor give you any advice?"

"Yes, he told me to eat whatever I wanted and to rest well."

Seeing I was puzzled with her answer, Ms. Wu continued, "They couldn't operate on me because I had heart problems and anemia. I would surely die on the operating table. Furthermore, I couldn't undergo chemotherapy because my body wouldn't take the strain. Imagine, even before I had cancer I needed to rest ten times in order to climb five flights of stairs. I was finished. But even facing death, I couldn't accept that my son would be a little orphan in the world.

"So I was desperate for a miracle. When someone mentioned that Chi Lel could help my condition, I immediately went to see a Chi-Lel master. He emitted chi to me and I responded well. I saw the light and took up Chi Lel. By the end of 1992 I was cured, and could climb five floors without resting or panting.

"When I returned to my doctor for a checkup, he was surprised to see me still alive. He confirmed that I was cancer free but said, 'If it disappeared by itself, it couldn't have been a cancer.' Yet at the same time he denied that he had misdiagnosed my case. I guess sometimes it's difficult to face facts when they are contradictory. But I don't care because either way I defeated a life-threatening illness.

"My whole family has taken up Chi Lel. By doing Chi Lel, my son's intelligence has improved. He has jumped from ranking as one of the last two students in his class to one of the top. Chi Lel is really wonderful."

23. The Most Stressful Job in China

"What illness have you recovered from, Teacher Zhou?"

"I was suffering from mental weakness. I couldn't concentrate on my work during the day and couldn't sleep at night. I was often angry at my family without reason and wasn't motivated to do anything at work. My supervisor understood my situation and was kind enough to let me off work very often. Neither Western nor Chinese medicine helped me at all, and I finally became so ineffectual at work that I was compelled to take a year off."

"What kind of work did you do?"

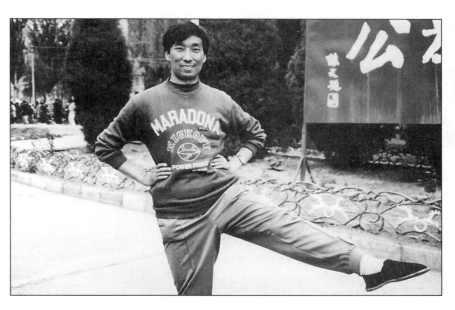

Zhou Shu-Zhi, 34, teacher

"I was a field agent responsible for carrying out our country's one-child policy. It is the most stressful job in China. Imagine telling a family in the countryside not to have another child when they have only a girl? But day in and day out, I had to confront one family after another. Stress built up over the years until I finally couldn't take it any longer."

"So Chi Lel helped you to recover?"

"Naturally, after taking up Chi Lel, my appetite and energy returned, my temper was brought under control and I could sleep at night. But at first Chi Lel was not easy. I couldn't concentrate on the movements because my mind was so agitated, and my belief in Chi Lel waned when, after practicing for two months, nothing happened—no instant improvements in my situation and no feeling of chi.

"I was almost to the point of giving up Chi Lel when my teacher suggested I practice with a group. 'With the collective chi effect of all the participants, you will concentrate more easily,' he assured me. I followed his advice and began to attend group practice sessions. Slowly I started to feel chi and that was enough to give me the confidence to come to the Center last year for three months of training. It was here that I finally found the promised benefits of Chi Lel. Now I have much tolerance for stress."

"Do you want to have your old job back?"

"No way! I'm through with that!"

I don't blame him for not wanting to test his newfound tolerance—would you?

24. We Dug Up Our Ancestors's Graves

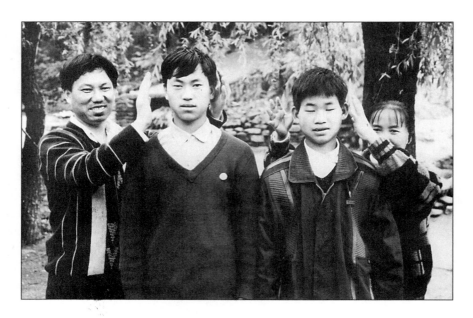

Zhang Zhi-Chong(r),16, Zhang Zhi-Biao, 18, with parents

"Can you hear me?" I asked the boy, Zhang Zhi-Chong, who was smiling from ear to ear.

"Yes," the boy replied. However, his mother quickly interrupted, "He can hear you, but he can't speak clearly because he's just started to develop language skills."

"What do you mean?"

"My son lost his hearing when he was two years old after a doctor treated his high fever. Unfortunately, he was not the only one; his brother also met the same fate. Of our four children, only my two girls have had normal hearing."

"Have you taken them to see specialists?"

"Yes, for the past ten years my husband and I have brought the boys to different hospitals all over the country for treatment, but to no avail. I have cried almost every day, asking 'Why the boys?' We even dug up our ancestors' graves to see if something was wrong with their burials. But nothing helped.

"Then one day a neighbor told us that their son's cancer had been cured by Chi Lel and strongly recommended that we go to the Center. Naturally, we brought our sons here immediately.

"It happened during the opening ceremony when Lao-shi shook hands with all the students. After shaking hands with Lao-shi, my younger son jumped with joy and gestured to me that he could hear! Tears came to my eyes. After so many years of agony and wait, finally my younger son could actually hear!"

"Do your sons take Chi Lel seriously?"

"Yes, both my sons religiously practice Chi Lel daily. My younger son's hearing is now normal and my older son's hearing, has also begun to improve, though less dramatically. From my heart I say thank you to Chi Lel. Long live Lao-shi!"

In fact, I had inadvertently videotaped the moment when Lao-shi shook hands with the younger son. Without realizing it, I had witnessed a miracle.

25. Can You See Through My Body?

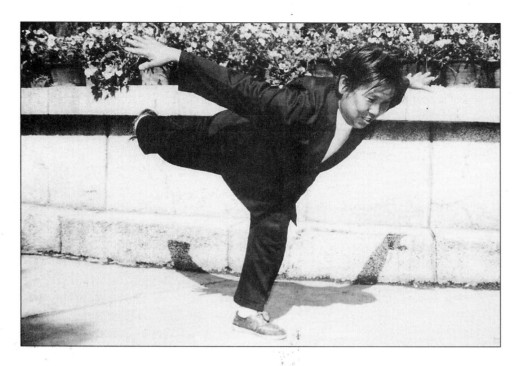

Ho Shu-Lan, 63, teacher

I had heard of certain talented individuals who have the ability to see through people, but I had never met one until now. Suppressing my eagerness to ask Teacher Ho about her talent at the beginning of the interview, I let her tell me her story.

"In 1958, I was afflicted with arthritis. All my joints became swollen and I could hardly walk. I took drugs every day just to be able to barely move. This was in addition to already, for twenty years, having high blood pressure and heart problems. My mind was becoming continuously confused and I was bordering on mental illness.

"The worst happened in 1985 when I had a life-threatening six-hour seizure. After that, I became paranoid and was always accusing people, especially my stepmother, of saying bad things about me behind my back. Indeed, my life was totally out of control.

"Luckily, a family friend saw my predicament and suggested Chi-Lel therapy. So in April 1988 I began learning Chi Lel near our home. I was attracted to it from the very first lesson and responded to chi very well. Even though at times lots of blood came out with my bowel movements and my pain increased, I kept on practicing Chi Lel.

"One night I couldn't breathe through my nose so I opened my mouth to breathe all night. When I woke up the next morning my nose had cleared and some pus was coming out of it. All my physical discomforts were gone. Then when I tried to look at my nose I saw something like a mirror in between my eyes. I looked inward and found strange red vessels. When I went to class and told my teacher what I had seen, he said excitedly, 'Congratulations! You have developed the 'see-through' ability. You probably saw the blood vessels of your brain.'

"Later, at home, I saw through my own body again and realized the teacher was right. At first people didn't believe I could see through their bodies, but as I would tell them their illnesses without asking, they began to believe. Later doctors in a hospital tested my ability by asking me to identify those women who were pregnant from among a group of patients. When my answers were right, they were convinced."

"So you can see through people like an X-ray machine. But what is the use of it?"

"Not much at first, until Lao-shi came to our city and saw me. He suggested that I use this special talent to heal the sick. Following his advice, I began my journey as a healer. The first case I worked on was a man with a broken arm. I saw through his broken bone and directed it to fuse again—and it worked!"

"How about your own health?"

"I was cured both physically and mentally many years ago. I have been a teacher here since 1991."

"Can you see chi?"

"Sure, I can see the chi around each internal organ of a person."

"Can you see through me and tell me if I am well?"

Teacher Ho nodded and closed her eyes for a minute. While she was doing that, I didn't feel any beams of energy going through my body. In fact, I didn't feel anything at all except a little bit worried, like someone waiting for the results of his physical checkup.

Finally Teacher Ho opened her eyes and with a smile said, "You are okay."

What a relief!

26. I Would Rather Die Dancing

I had noticed Ms. Yang even before interviewing her—she was an attractive lady with sandy blond hair among a homogeneous black-haired crowd. I thought she must be the child of a mixed marriage, coming from a Chinese-Russian boarder city. But she wasn't.

"Last March I started to bleed not only during my period but also at other times too. The bleeding was accompanied by abdominal pain. My mother took me to the hospital for a checkup. I didn't think anything serious could happen to a young person like me and my mother also reassured me. But she told me I needed to go to the hospital for some routine treatment.

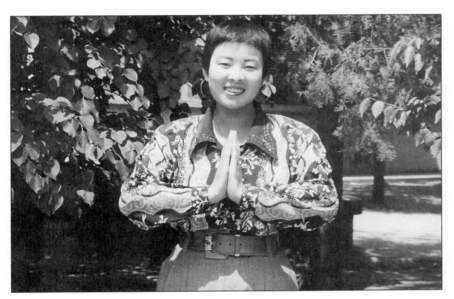

Yang Gui-Chong, 24, student

"In the hospital, they hooked me up to a bottle of liquid and began to deliver its contents into my veins. It was very painful but my mother told me that the doctors did this routinely in bleeding cases. While before I was a very active girl, now I was bound to the bed, watching liquid going into my body drop by drop. I even counted its rate—one minute for every seventeen drops. It would take forever for the bottle to empty!

"My boy friend and his mother came to see me often. They were so nice to me that I became suspicious. Why was it that each time they left, they behaved as if they would never see me again? That bad? When my hair started to fall out and my stay in the hospital was prolonged, I began to realize that I was indeed in serious trouble. I found out I had uterine cancer! My young life would be over in three years unless I responded to the chemotherapy or surgery."

"I heard it's expensive to have surgery done. Could your family have afforded it?"

"Money is not an issue for my family. My father owns two karaoke cafes and I love to dance there. During chemotherapy, my parents wanted to keep me from crowded places because they were afraid that I would pick up germs. So when I donned a wig and showed up at one of their cafes, my mother was startled and ordered me to leave at once. I didn't budge and told her I would rather die dancing. I danced the night away, forgetting my troubles.

"Yet my troubles didn't go away. I was told that chemotherapy was not helping me and that surgically removing my uterus remained as the only option. What kind of option is that? Even if cured I would be a woman without a uterus. I was chilled at the thought of being incapable of bearing children.

"The day before they sent me to the best hospital in Beijing for the operation, I was very depressed and didn't want to go. Then my mother asked offhandedly if I wanted to try Chi Lel.

Beaming with delight, I replied with a resounding yes even though I didn't know what I was getting into."

"Why did your mother suggest Chi Lel to you?"

"By coincidence, my mother had talked to someone about my situation who happened to have a relative recovering from leukemia in the Center. My mother was not at all convinced about Chi Lel and was afraid it would be a false hope for me. But seeing me so enthusiastic about going to the Center, she brought me to see the former leukemia patient. By talking to a person who had actually recovered from cancer, I began to believe with my heart and soul that my cancer too, could be cured with Chi Lel. So with that hope I came here two months ago.

"I studied Chi Lel seriously, getting up early in the morning and going to bed late. Every day I did an extra hour and a half of the Wall Squatting exercise, plus everything else my teacher told me to do. After ten days my abdomen began to hurt even more. 'Good, pain is good,' my teacher told me. But after the first month, the doctors told me that my tumor had actually become bigger than before! Being more puzzled than afraid, I asked my teacher what was going on. 'Sometimes chi balloons up a tumor, it will go away,' he replied.

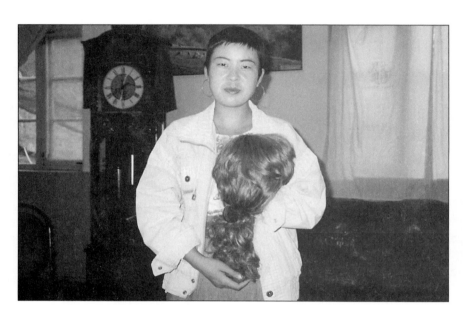

Ms. Yang takes off her wig

"I worked even harder. A month later when I went in for another checkup, I was told that my cancer was gone! Gone! Gone!"

"So you can go home and dance now."

"Actually, I would rather go home and practice Chi Lel. Instead of throwing money away eating and having fun I would rather donate it to the Center so that more people like myself can be helped."

"That's very kind of you, Ms. Young. I have a request. May I see your real hair?"

She took off her wig, revealing her real hair, short but beautiful. I took a picture of her and commented that her hair was pretty just as it was. I never saw her wearing her unnaturally colored wig again.

27. I Gave Money Away

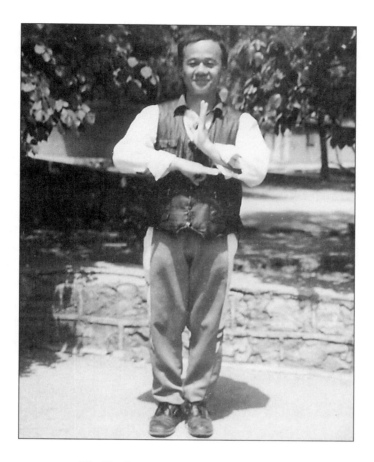

Hu Fu-Lin, 45, instructor trainee

Mr. Fu is a short man, no more than five feet tall, with a bald forehead and a baby face. He doesn't look his age.

"After working on a stressful project day and night for a week in 1992, my body and mind collapsed. I couldn't sleep at night, had severe headaches, and developed a rapid heart rate. At times I lost my mind. So I ended up being hospitalized for more than half a year."

"What do you mean by losing your mind?"

"Sometimes I wouldn't know what was going on around me. I even gave money away without knowing it. After my hospitalization, I went back to work but couldn't concentrate on my job. I felt depressed, thinking my life was finished.

"Luckily, I knew of a neighbor who had been cured by Chi Lel. Seeing is believing: I reasoned that if Chi Lel was effective against cancer it would be good for me too. So I took up Chi Lel. Within three months, all my symptoms were gone. I have never felt better in my life."

"Are you still giving money away?"

"No way, sir!"

28. I Was An Old Man at 25 and A Young Man at 52

Since childhood Mr. Wang had suffered poor health. With his pale face and thin body, even in his early twenties people already addressed him as "old man."

"My heart would sometimes beat rapidly without reason, and I had severe headaches and stomach ailments. Then came arthritis. All the joints of my body were affected and I was immobilized in the hospital for months. When my doctor gave me a bunch of pills to help me sleep, I used them to attempt suicide. But it didn't work, I woke up still in hell."

"Why did you want to end your life?"

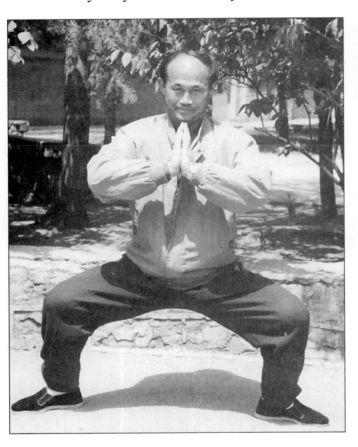

Wang Li-Hua, 53, instructor trainee

"Why? The excruciating pain! I could only sleep a few minutes at a time because of it. Life was very, very miserable for me. Later I tried to commit suicide again but again I was saved. Finally, I gave up trying to kill myself, preferring to endure life as best I could."

"So when did you start Chi Lel?"

"In 1988, a doctor told me that I would become blind within one year because the blood vessels in my eyes were hardening. I panicked and started looking for miracles. It happened that Lao-shi was in town giving a lecture on Chi Lel and I attended and learned the self-healing art. After practicing Chi Lel for a year, all my illnesses are gone and I can still see. Moreover, people have begun to call me big brother instead of old man. So I was an old man at twenty-five and a young man at fifty-two." Mr. Wang laughed and continued,"To repay what Chi Lel has given me, I've become very active in promoting the art. I am the vice president of our province's Chi-Lel association, which has 20,000 members."

"How does your organization measure a teacher's effectiveness?"

"We measure a teacher's effectiveness by the number of students he has taught and by the number of patients he has successfully helped to heal."

"Are you an effective teacher?"

Upon hearing my question, Mr. Wang took several photos out of his pocket to show me some difficult cases with which he'd helped. One picture showed a woman in a hospital with Mr. Wang emitting chi to her. He told me that he had saved the dying woman. Another two photos were before and after pictures of a young disabled girl who had undergone Chi-Lel therapy. In the first one, saliva is dripping from her mouth, while in the other she is smiling, with much better control over her body.

Maybe the reason Mr. Wang was saved twice from killing himself is that he has been chosen to become a savior himself?

29. I'll Write to You, But Please Don't Reply

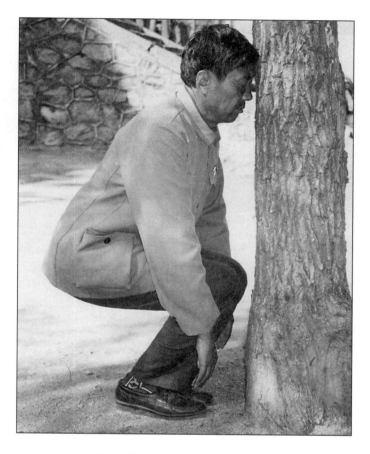

Sun Sheng-Mo, 49, student

When Mr. Sun was diagnosed with stomach cancer last October, he didn't want his family to know. Surgery was suggested but he wanted to wait until after the new year.

"On New Year's Day, a friend, who had learned of my situation asked me to join his Chi-Lel group, saying 'surgery is not a guarantee of success, why not try Chi Lel?' So I joined his group for two months and then came here."

"Were you still thinking about surgery while you were doing Chi Lel?"

"Well, surgery was one alternative. But put it this way, with my life at stake, I would have tried anything that worked. While I felt Chi Lel was a better choice for me, I knew that, in order for chi to work on me, I must have absolute belief and dedication.

"So before I left for the Center, I gathered my wife and children together and told them, 'I'll write to you, but please don't reply. I don't want to be bothered with anything.'

"During the next three months, I wrote four letters to my family, each letter bearing better news than the previous one. A short time later, my cancer totally disappeared.

"Did you work hard?"

"Absolutely, I did my Chi Lel at four o'clock every morning before anyone woke up. Even with a high fever, I still did the Wall-Squatting exercise two hundred and ten times."

"Weren't you afraid that your condition was getting worse when you had the fever?"

"I believed my fever was a reaction to the healing chi, and so it was good."

30. I Had Been Waiting Forty Years

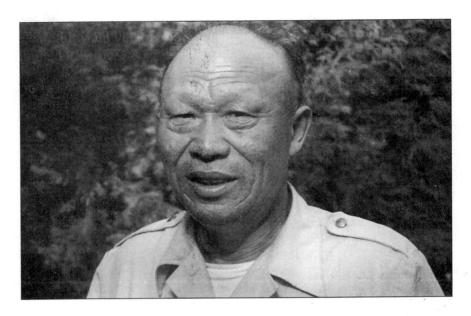

Xu Cheng-Run, 58, instructor trainee

Before taking up Chi Lel, Mr. Xu could only sleep two to three hours each night because he had arteriosclerosis in some of the blood vessels that supply oxygen to his brain. In addition, he had high blood pressure and diabetes, and took different medications daily for these ailments.

"The drugs were expensive and troublesome and I couldn't go anywhere without them. Yet they provided only some relief, without actually curing any of my illnesses. My body was becoming weaker each day. Then last October a friend recommended Chi Lel and I joined a local group. Within two months, I didn't need to take medications anymore, and my body weight returned to normal. I gained thirty-four pounds."

"Why do you want to take the three-month instructor's course?"

"I want to solidify my gains and learn more about Chi Lel. While I was here, a small miracle had happened to me."

"What miracle?"

"My face cleared up!"

When I couldn't understand what he was talking about, Mr. Xu pointed to his face.

"You mean acne? I thought that only occurred in young people and then later disappeared."

"Yes, but I've been waiting forty years for it to disappear," Mr. Xu shook his head. "I've been ugly all my life."

"Congratulations, you are a handsome man now!" Mr. Xu smiled like a teenager and I continued,"Be careful when you get home, your wife might attack you!"

We both laughed heartily.

31. Please Don't Laugh at Me

For thirteen years, Ms. Li walked on crutches, mostly confined to bed.

"My paralysis was caused by drug poisoning. Even though I was hospitalized for three years, still the doctors couldn't do anything for me. At home, I would sit in my bed most of the time, waiting for others to serve me."

"Could you move around?"

"Very little. My feet felt numb as though I were walking on cotton. My right shoulder and back were pressed together as a result of walking on crutches. My internal organs were not functioning well due to lack of proper movement. Indeed, at the prime of my life, I had become a liability for my family. I longed for a miracle that would free me.

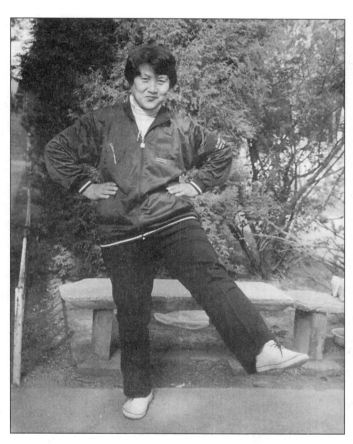

Li Xiang-Rong, 58, instructor trainee

"Then one day in 1986 I read Laoshi's book on Chi Lel. From his book, I learned the simple movements to deliver chi to myself. Yet the idea that I could improve my condition or even to stop being a cripple was unthinkable. People would think I was crazy. So I kept Chi Lel a secret. I begged people silently not to laugh at me for trying to do the unthinkable.

"After two years of practicing the movements alone, my condition improved enough so that I could walk around my house with a stick. When I could finally walk to the park, I joined the Chi-Lel class that met there.

"On my first day, the teacher, surprised to find I had a lot of chi, asked 'You've just started, how can you do the movements so well?'

"When I told her my story, she embraced me and told me that I was finally home. With this sympathetic group, improvements were immediate. I accomplished more in two months than in the years I had spent practicing alone. Now I can walk freely and my body has regained its original form. Indeed, I have better health than the average person. My dream has finally become a reality, and I am free at last!"

I thanked Ms. Li for sharing her story with me. At the same time, I wondered how many people in this world are being laughed for daring to do the "unthinkable," bringing miracles to themselves.

32. Let's Face It, You Are Too Old for Anything

After suffering a stroke in 1982, Ms. Chi lost the ability to take care of herself. She couldn't walk without assistance, and her hands were useless, unable to hold a rice bowl or a pair of chopsticks. Even when going to the bathroom, she needed her daughter to untie her trousers. She was totally dependent.

"Did you give up hope?"

"No, with my family's help, I went to different hospitals for treatment. But none could help me. Then I became depressed when I overheard a doctor telling my son, 'Let's face it. She is too old for anything. She should be happy where she is.'"

"Did you want to end you life?"

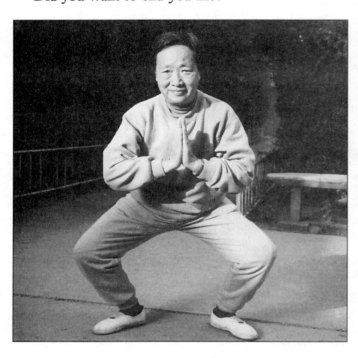

Chi Ji-Xun, 72, instructor trainee

"No, I still hoped that one day there would be new drugs for my illnesses. So I waited. In fact I waited eight years. My body deteriorated to the point where I couldn't see or hear clearly, and my house became a virtual prison.

"Then one day someone told me that Chi Lel could be helpful for my condition. That was the only encouragement I'd had in eight years and I wanted to try the therapy immediately. So my son carried me to the train, and my daughter and I left for the Center. After half a month in the Center, I was well enough that my daughter could go home."

"Was it easy for you to go through the Chi-Lel program?"

"It was hard but joyful. When I first saw people in wheelchairs beginning to walk, I believed that I could overcome my infirmities too. I worked very hard. Unable to stand freely, I balanced against a tree to do the Chi-Lel movements. Even with the tree I fell countless times.

"After fifty days all my ailments were gone, and I could do the movements without the help of trees. Now I come back to the Center once a year to sharpen my Chi-Lel skill. At home, I can take care of my son and daughter instead of them taking care of me."

"Are you glad you have taken up Chi Lel?"

"Certainly, but with one regret."

"What's that?"

"I wish I had learned it when I was younger."

"But you are still young."

With a smile, she replied, "That's true, my teacher told me that when we practice Chi Lel, we are not senior citizens until the age of ninety-five."

33. It Was a Minor Problem

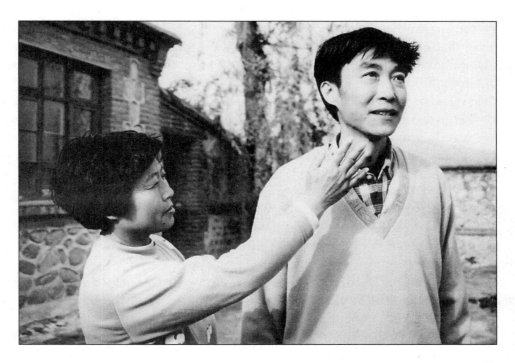

Lu Pei-De, 52, student, with teacher

Mr. Lu, a high school teacher and newspaper reporter, had lung cancer in 1991. After having his right lung surgically removed and undergoing chemotherapy for a year and half, his cancer temporarily went into remission.

"Being a reporter, I have in the past been very active in encouraging people with cancer to promptly undergo surgery and chemotherapy. In fact, I was elected secretary of the Cancer Society of Shanghai."

"Were you aware of Chi Lel at the time?"

"No, there are many types of qigong in Shanghai, and I have never paid too much attention to them. I didn't believe in their healing power."

"What made you change your mind?"

"When two cancerous lumps reappeared on my neck two years later, doctors were unable to help me. They told me that I was too weak to undergo another surgery and put me on chemotherapy for a few months. When chemotherapy didn't help, I was on my own. I had reached a dead end, and I was ready for anything.

"It so happened that at this time Lao-shi was giving a lecture in Shanghai, and I was given a ticket to see him. Even though I felt very weak, I managed, with the help of a taxi, to get to the lecture. Just from listening to Lao-shi's talk, my energy level increased enough for me to go home on a crowded bus. When I got home I began to eat as though I had been hungry for a long time. Indeed, my appetite had returned; I asked my wife, 'Why is everything so sweet and tasty?'

"With new hope, my wife and I arrived at the Center in November 1994. When I told my teacher why I had come to the Center, she asked me to show her the lumps on my neck. 'This is a minor problem,' she said, delivering chi to my neck. 'Touch them to see if they have disappeared.'

"Unbelievably, my lumps were gone! My wife touched my neck and couldn't find them either—the lumps were gone!

"Seeing that my lumps had disappeared, my wife asked, 'Teacher, I also have a lump on my neck, would you fix it for me?' 'No problem,' our teacher replied, delivering chi. My wife's benign tumor also left in an instant!

"While we were jumping for joy, I realized that my chest no longer hurt when I laughed. Later when I went to see my doctors, they were unable to believe what they were seeing for themselves. But that was their problem."

To prove his point, Mr. Lu showed me his neck, and I could find no trace of any tumors.

I asked the teacher why some people have instant results while others take a long time to heal.

The teacher replied, "Each person reacts differently to chi. In the Center, we have built up a large healing chi-field. Mr. Lu and his wife are very sensitive to our chi. It was not my own power that had cured their tumors, but the combination of their willingness to open themselves up to chi healing and the healing effect of our environment. I was only a medium for this interaction."

No one at the Center claims to have magical power. Chi Lel is treated as a science which needs to be studied. The hope is that the more the behavior of chi is understood, the more we can use it to make our lives better.

34. Partner, I'll Take Care of You for the Next Thirty Years

At the age of twenty-seven, Ms. Hao, a mother of three, suddenly developed heart disease and arthritis. With disabled legs and a delicate heart, she spent the next decade at home, relying on daily doses of medicine to relieve pain.

When her illnesses stabilized, she returned to work on crutches. Then, in 1982, her heart gave out all together and she underwent heart surgery. Following that, her heart functioned normally and it was nine years before she again had a problem.

"In 1992 I lost my appetite, and started to feel a different type of pain. At first I ignored these symptoms because I was used to pain but a few months later doctors told me that my gallbladder was filled with stones. They couldn't do anything about this condition because my gallbladder didn't have enough juice inside it. I asked if they could operate on me, but they said I couldn't

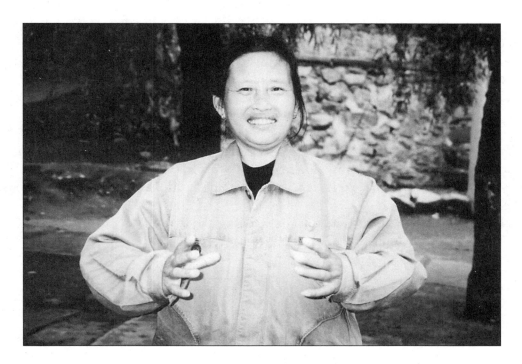

Hao Ying-Jie, 54, student

stand another operation because of my heart condition. So I had no other option left but to bear my pain and wait to die.

"Then a friend came to see me and told me that a friend of hers had recovered from heart disease using Chi Lel. I grasped this good news like someone holding on to a lifesaver in the open sea, and, persuading my husband to come with me, I left for the Center on the first available train. When I encountered my doctor on the way to the railway station, he jeered, saying, 'Chi Lel? I'll bet you five hundred yuan it won't work.' I replied, 'I raise your bet to a thousand yuans that I will come back healthy.'

"When I reached the Center, I felt at home at once. The minute I saw my teacher, he asked, 'Are you tired after such a long journey?' 'No,' I replied. 'Good, then come and do the Chi Lel

41

now!' he said, leading me to our group. So I haven't lost a moment of practice time since I arrived here.

"I practiced Chi Lel very diligently. Even though I had a high fever for four days after shaking hands with Lao-shi, I welcomed it as good news because I knew that chi was working on me."

"How did you know that the fever was a response to chi?"

"If it were an ordinary fever, my spirit wouldn't have been high and my appetite wouldn't have been good. Besides, I was so convinced that chi was working on me that my thoughts alone would have easily turned a bad fever into a good one.

"In less than a month after I was here, my gallbladder was cleared of stones. Look," Ms. Hao took out a small bottle of stones from her pocket and continued, "I've been collecting them as souvenirs."

"What was your husband's reaction?"

"Of course he is very happy. I have become younger looking as my heart disease and other illnesses have disappeared. I asked him to go home because I am now able to take care of myself. Before he went, however, I said to him, 'Partner, you have been taking care of me for the past twenty-seven years; now it is my turn to take care of you for the next thirty years.'"

"Can you share what went through your mind when you did your Chi Lel?"

"Yes, of course. When doing the standing method, I imagined my gallbladder opening to the universe and then closing in to gather chi. While doing La Chi (opening and closing of hands) I imagined my entire body disappearing into infinity. I actually felt that I had become a mass of chi with no physical body. One day, while doing the standing method, I prayed to Lao-shi: 'Lao-shi, I know that you are very busy now, but please give me some attention. My name is Hao Ying-Jie, and I'm a healthy person now—*Wan Yuan Lin Toon* (Chi is Omnipotent).'"

"Thank you, Ms. Hao. One more question: Are you going to ask your doctor for the thousand yuans?"

"Sure, I'll ask him for the money and then donate it to the Center."

Ms. Hao bet her life and won.

35. Unexpectedly My Child Stood Up

"Just after I was married in 1979, my health declined rapidly. First, I developed stomach trouble, then I had problems with my liver, and finally my lungs went bad. Two years later, while I was still struggling with my health, our son was born. This gave me much joy. But the joy didn't last long because soon a dentist noticed a small bean-sized growth in my son's upper lip. I took him to see a doctor who told me that my son had a blood vessel tumor.

"This type of tumor normally isn't a serious threat to one's health, but for my son the tumor was a major problem since it was located in a place where surgery couldn't be performed. As the tumor steadily swelled, I brought my son to different hospitals in various large cities for treatment. Doctors tried different methods including freezing the tumor and using electric shocks; however, rather than helping, these treatments actually stimulated the tumor's growth. I saw my

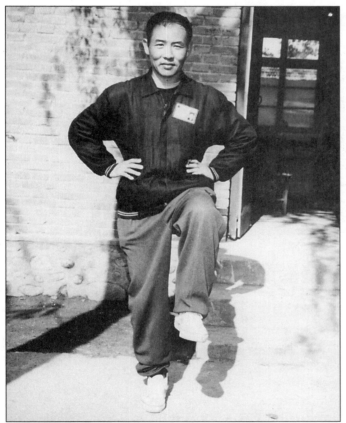

Jing Shan, 46, teacher

child's lip being pushed up towards his nose every day, and I was worried to death."

"What about your own health?"

"I lost interest in my own health. When doctors discovered a cancerous spot on my skin, I didn't even care. Cancer or no cancer, what difference would it make if my child died?

"When my child was ten years old, his tumor grew so much that it almost blocked his nose. My heart sank each time I saw him gasping for air. The doctors predicted he had only six months to live.

"A shroud of sadness covered our family. We were helplessly watching our child gradually choking to death. When a friend suggested we try Chi Lel, we were in no mood to listen. If all these prestigious hospitals with all their experts couldn't cure our son, what could Chi Lel do? I thanked our friend, but dismissed his idea as wishful thinking and an attempt to comfort us."

"Why did you think this way?"

"Well, in a hospital, I can see the knives, the pills, the needles, and the fluids and I can smell the sanitary agents and different types of drugs. But Chi Lel? I couldn't see, smell, or hear chi. It was unreal to me at the time."

"What happened next?"

"The friend, who was a Chi -Lel practitioner, kept on encouraging me to take the self-healing art, saying, 'What if Chi Lel works? You owe it to your son to try it.' My friend's sincerity and unwavering belief in Chi Lel gradually softened my heart and finally dispelled any last hope I had in modern medicine. Embracing Chi Lel as the only hope of curing of my son's condition, I brought him to the Center.

"After twenty-four days of Chi Lel, my son's tumor not only stopped growing but also began to shrink. Furthermore, my own health had improved to the point that I could ride a bicycle! The climax of our visit occurred during a lecture by Lao-shi in which he asked people to stand up if they had tumors which had softened, become smaller, or disappeared. I saw my son stand up. I couldn't believe my eyes, his tumor was gone! My ten-year-old's tumor was gone! I thought I was in a dream. But when I touched my son, it was real. His tumor had gone! Tears rushed to my eyes."

"Did the tumor just disappear like that, instantly?"

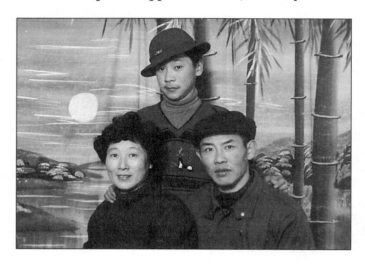

Teacher Jing with his wife and son

"Just like that."

"Did it ever come back?"

"It came back as a tiny spot but never grew any bigger. It eventually left my son entirely. After the miracle, my health, too, completely recovered."

"During your recoveries, did you both work hard?"

"Absolutely. We did a lot of Wall Squatting. My son's record was 700 times in a row."

"That's incredible."

With a smile, Teacher Jing added, "My record was 1,200."

"Can you show us how to do the Wall Squatting exercise?"

"Sure," Teacher Jing replied and demonstrated the exercise in front of a wall. I took some pictures of him doing the Wall Squatting (See Wall Squatting in Part Two of this book).

"What's your son doing now and why are you here?"

"He is seventeen now, a healthy high-school boy. I have become a teacher at the Center so that I can help people who are now in the same shoes as we were. Also, I send chi to my family every day."

Teacher Jing talked of sending chi as matter-of-factly as he did a letter. What a change from being a "logical" person who only trusted his five senses.

36. Healing Others, Healing Herself

This is the story of Ms. Chiao who, along with practicing Chi Lel, took a different route to recovery.

"After the birth of my son in 1977, my joints began to show symptoms of arthritis. In addition, my spleen and liver were enlarged, I had heart problems, and I began to have severe headaches. These ailments, together with the asthma I'd had for thirty-two years, rendered me a virtually useless person.

"Moreover, my family was in discord, which created a lot of stress. Finally, my mind just gave out. I would cry one moment and laugh the next; sometimes I wanted to hit people."

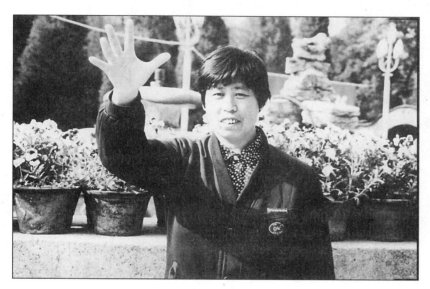

Chiao Zuo-Xian, 44, teacher

"Did you go to the hospital?"

"Yes, but doctors couldn't do much and I relied on daily medications to live. I asked myself, if doctors can't help me and my family doesn't love me, what kind of life is this? So I took an overdose of sleeping pills to kill myself. When I woke up, I realized I was in hell. In addition to all my other problems, the sleeping pills had damaged my stomach. For the next eight years, I had to endure the pain of all my ailments without relief because my stomach could no longer absorb any medication."

"When did you begin Chi Lel?"

"When Lao-shi came to our city in 1988. I wanted badly to see him because I had heard wondrous things about Chi Lel, but my husband adamantly opposed my going. He dismissed Chi Lel as phony, saying it only appeals to gullible people and those who have lost their minds."

"Couldn't you have gone by yourself?"

With a choking voice, she replied, "I couldn't walk. I needed his help."

"Did he finally help you?"

"Not until I protested with a seizure. My convulsions remained out of control until my husband agreed to carry me to the auditorium.

"After attending Lao-shi's lecture, my heart and soul opened, and when I joined our Chi-Lel group, I was able to walk there by myself. In fact, from the first day of Chi Lel, I began to heal others."

"Healing others? Were all your illnesses gone?"

"Not yet, I was still suffering from my infirmities. However, I had an urge to help others and behaved as if I were already a healthy person. I practiced Chi Lel diligently during the day and healed others at night, without charging them a penny. Gradually, I became well known in our area as an effective healer. Meanwhile, all my illnesses disappeared without me paying much attention to them."

"Was your husband supportive of what you were doing?"

"Not until I cured his mental depression, my son's eyesight, and my daughter's headaches."

"Can you share with us how you facilitate healing?"

"Each time I perform a healing, I imagine that my hand has become Lao-shi's hand and he is delivering chi to me and the patient."

By healing others, Teacher Chiao also healed herself.

37. Teased by His Classmates

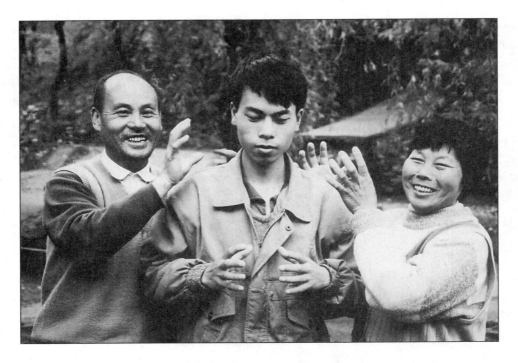

Liu Xing-Ceng, 21, student, with parents

At first I couldn't comprehend in medical terms how bad Mr. Liu's hearing was, but then I understood when he said, "I couldn't even hear the school bell ring."

He went on to tell me that he had tried many treatments, including putting special electrically charged acupuncture needles in his ears. "It was very painful, and it didn't help."

"When did you start Chi Lel?"

"In early 1994, my high school teacher taught me the Chi-Lel movement La Chi (opening and closing the hands). After practicing the movement about four hours a day for fourteen days, my ears started to hurt very much. But as I continued to practice the pain disappeared and my hearing improved. My teacher was overjoyed and became zealous about spreading Chi Lel, using me as a model to demonstrate how Chi Lel could help people.

"The kids in school, however, instead of learning Chi Lel, started to tease me. When I told them that I could feel chi they said I was crazy, and, since they kept bothering me, I couldn't concentrate on Chi Lel anymore. I quit practicing and so lost my hearing again.

"Then a year later, after trying other fruitless treatments, my parents decided to bring me to the Center. With encouragement from the Chi-Lel teachers, I started to do the Chi Lel again, and now hear clearly."

"Do you feel safe in the Center?"

"Yes, I feel very much at home here because no one teases me. If believing and feeling chi is crazy, then at the Center we are all insane."

38. Say Farewell to the Great Wall

After giving Mr. Shu a routine physical examination in August of 1994, doctors had bad news for him. But he wasn't to know the truth about his condition until much later.

"After the checkup, my wife suddenly became very attentive to me, granting me my every wish. She even suggested that we visit the Great Wall, a place I had always wanted to go, adding, 'I've heard that there is a place near Beijing where people can heal their illnesses.'

"I replied, 'Dear, you told me that I would recover soon. Why should I go to a place a thousand miles away to heal myself?' But my wife insisted that our trip was mainly to see the Great Wall in our capital city, not for medical reasons."

"So did you go to the Great Wall?"

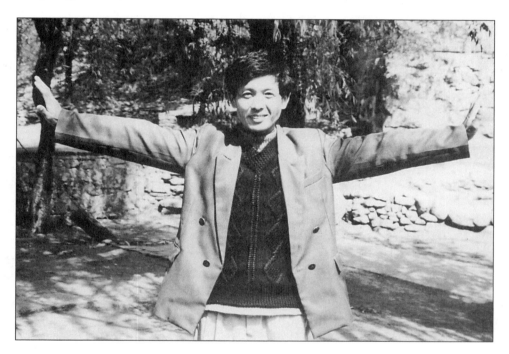

Shu Hai-Lin, 38, student

"Yes, but while on the Great Wall, instead of feeling exalted, I felt very weak and tired. Furthermore, I had almost no appetite. I began to wonder if the doctors had misdiagnosed my illness. I was happy when we finally were on a train to a place where I could find help.

"When we arrived at the Center, I felt very much at home. Although I was very tired, I kept up with the Chi-Lel schedule. Improvement was immediate; after three days, I began to eat and my strength returned to me. After reading one of Lao-shi's books, I became convinced that Chi Lel would help me and so took every Chi-Lel session seriously. Soon I felt chi around and inside me. I was on my way to recovery."

"Did you know your ailment by that time?"

"No. It wasn't until one day almost at the end of my 24-day Chi-Lel program when an instructor trainee, ignorant of my condition, was emitting chi to me. He showed me my doctor's diagnosis—liver cancer!"

47

"Were you shocked?"

"I was surprised to know my illness was so serious. But by that time, I was feeling so good that I believed my cancer had left me—or if not, would disappear sooner or later as long as I continued to practice Chi Lel.

"A few days later, I went to see a doctor who, using an ultrasound, couldn't find any trace of cancer in my liver. Even though the result was expected, I felt much relieved."

"What were you thinking when you did Chi Lel to get rid of your tumor?"

"I imagined my entire body disappearing into blue sky when opening, and when closing, imagined that life energy was gathering into a small tube going through my body's centerline from the top of my head to my groin. I felt no physical body, only life energy within."

I thanked Mr. Shu for sharing his experience with me and concluded the interview by asking, "What do you want to do when you pass through Beijing again?"

"See the Great Wall."

"I thought you'd already seen it."

"Yes. But I didn't have the strength to climb its steps."

With newfound energy, Mr. Shu was about to do what most people take for granted—climb some steps.

39. I Wouldn't Have Been Able Tell Whether You Were a Man Or a Woman

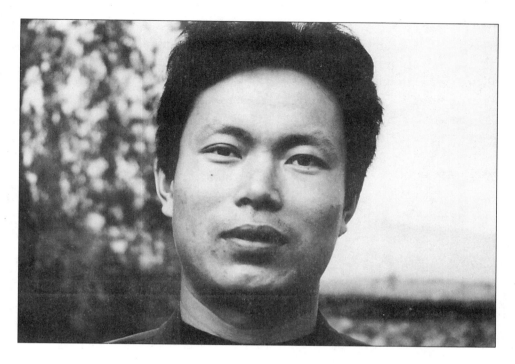

Shan Fu-Yau, 25, student

Mr. Shan told me that five years ago, on the day before his high school final examination, he suddenly became blind.

"Would you have been able to see me then?" I asked Mr. Shan, who was sitting across from me.

"Yes, but I wouldn't have been able to tell whether you were a man or a woman."

"Did you seek help from eye specialists?"

"Of course, I went to different hospitals and tried everything but nothing helped me regain my vision. Constantly afraid of light, my life became miserable. Then last month I encountered a friend who had been cured of lung cancer at the Center. I made up my mind to come here as a last hope.

"With the help of my teacher and other classmates, I settled down comfortably at the Center. Then a miracle happened. One day, while I was practicing Chi Lel with others, I suddenly saw the characters, Wan Yuan Ling Toon (Chi is Omnipotent) on a banner! It was the first time in five years that I could actually see. After that, my vision became better every day and now I am no longer afraid of light."

"Where do you want to go from here?"

"I want to join the Chi-Lel Academy and devote my life to the science of Chi Lel."

Another potential teacher in the making.

40. An Orange Saved a Professor's Life

Professor Meng told me that his family's roots can be traced back to the seventy-first generation of the famous scholar Meng Tse. Certainly he himself is a scholar in his own right. He is an expert in electronic communications, and at one time worked on a government satellite program.

"In 1992, I was diagnosed with lymphatic cancer. The cancer spread rapidly from my legs to my kidneys and then to my entire body. The doctors predicted that I had only three or four months to live. When my friends and students found out I was dying, many came to say good-bye to me. But I told them that I was not dead until I was dead."

"Why were you so brave?"

"It was not that I was brave but that I was a believer in miracles. Two years before, during the time I was with Lao-shi, an 'incurable' clot in a blood vessel in my brain was cured. This time, I had a faint hope that Lao-shi would again come to my rescue. So I sent him a letter. Since Lao-shi is very busy and always on the road, I wondered, if my letter would reach him in time.

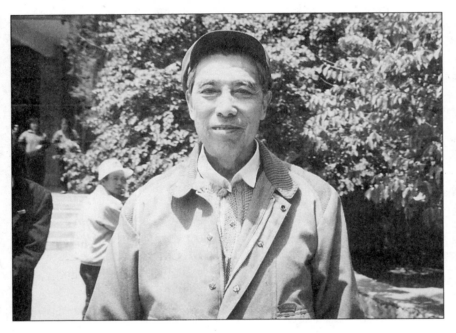

Meng Zhao-Chui, 71, head of the Center's Research Department

"Unexpectedly, I received an orange a few days later. It was from Lao-shi who just happened to have been passing by our city. Holding the orange in my hand, I uttered, 'I'm saved!' Then six Chi-Lel masters were sent to emit chi to me. When they found out I couldn't move much, they told me to continue practicing Chi Lel by using just my fingers and imagining myself opening to the universe and gathering chi into my body.

"Before they left, the leader told me, 'Miracles will happen; they must happen.' I truly believed his words. With new hope, I continued chemotherapy and the cancer was suppressed. However, during the next two years, the cancer returned and left three times. The last time it reappeared was almost a year ago."

"Professor Meng, as a top-notched scientist, how do you justify your belief in Chi Lel?"

"We scientists believe evidence and I approach Chi Lel the same way. Since my expertise is electronics, I've designed many experiments which investigate the effect of chi on electric phenomena. I've just finished an experiment where chi was emitted to dead batteries, and they were recharged. Besides doing experiments on my own, I'm also a liaison for many universities that are conducting experiments with the Center. By the way, before you leave for America, I'll give you some information about our experiments."

A few days later, Professor Meng gave me two volumes of data from experiments they had done—both almost as thick as a telephone book!

41. An Acupuncturist Became a "Barehanded Doctor"

Dr. Chao, an acupuncturist, was forced into retirement at the age of fifty-two because of disabling illnesses.

"I had very low blood pressure, which caused me to faint frequently. My lungs were not functioning properly and I often vomited blood. I had stomachaches, chest pain, and a hernia.

"My son and son-in-law, both trained in Western medicine, couldn't help me and my own acupuncture didn't help either. At age fifty-two, I was merely vegetating at home, waiting for heaven to take me. Being a practical man, I made no attempt to seek an alternative way out of my plight. So when a friend mentioned Chi Lel to me, I dismissed it as wishful thinking."

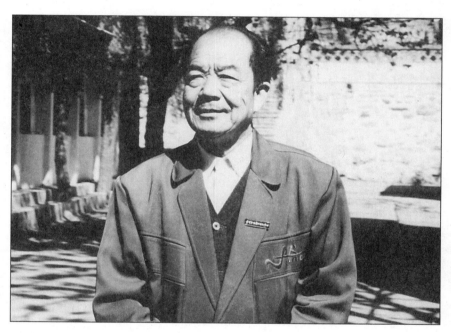

Chao Hai-Chao, 62, teacher

"Why? I thought you would believe in chi since you were an acupuncturist."

"Well, I used needles to heal people. But if Chi Lel actually heals people, what good are needles?

"Nevertheless, my wife became interested in Chi Lel."

"Why did your wife become interested?"

"Because she had both an open mind and a need. For many years, she could only sleep two hours at a time and ate very little. After a few days of Chi Lel, I saw the transformation of my wife—her appetite returned and she could sleep soundly. Seeing her change, I plunged into Chi Lel with all my heart and soul.

"I read many of Lao-shi's books and practiced Chi Lel day and night, getting so involved that I even forgot to take my daily medicine. After a few days, my blood pressure had risen slightly and I was no longer vomiting blood. A month later, my blood pressure had returned to normal and my chest pain disappeared. After one year, my lungs also healed. I was a new person all over again."

"Did you go back to practicing acupuncture?"

"No way. I went to the Center for a three-month training and am now a Chi-Lel teacher. I've taught more than ten thousand students. In addition, I've led volunteers into remote villages to teach people Chi Lel. Because we charge very little money, many of these patients would not otherwise have been able to afford medical treatment, and, because of their strong belief in our method, the healing rate was astonishing. I personally healed many people with kidney and gallbladder stones, diabetes, and many other chronic diseases."

"So you are sort of "barefoot doctors," sacrificing personal comfort to serve the sick?"

"We're more than barefoot doctors—we are barehanded doctors who use no medicines at all in our treatments!"

42. I Ate a Lot of Rice

In 1986, Teacher Zhou, at the age of forty-nine, was so sick that she was forced to take an early retirement. Her heart would beat rapidly after just taking a few steps; she had severe headaches, an ovarian tumor, and a tendency to faint while walking on the street.

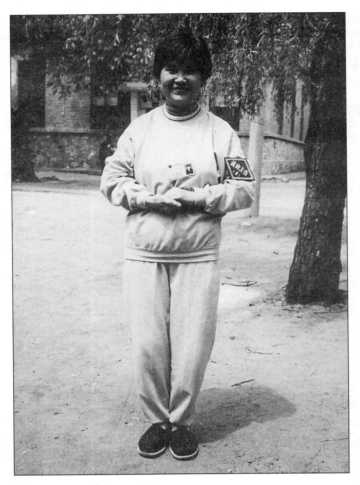

Zhou Fu-Chin, 58, teacher

"Although I ate a lot of rice, I still had no strength. The doctors told me it had something to do with my glandular system not working properly. So without any strength to walk, I was confined to bed, waiting helplessly for my organs to fail. Indeed, life was nothing but suffering.

"Then one day, a friend mentioned Chi Lel and asked me to join their group. But I wasn't interested."

"Why not? You had nothing to lose."

"I had tried other types of qigong before and they didn't work for me. Why would I waste my time now?

"Yet my friend persisted, visiting me often and emitting chi to me every time. My resistance melted as I felt better after receiving chi from my friend. So I joined her Chi-Lel group. With encouragement from my friend and other members of the group, I gradually regained my strength. By 1993 I was able to come to the Center by myself to study. One day, during Lao-shi's lecture, I discovered a lot of water coming out of my big toes. Intuitively, I knew my tumor was dissolving, and this was later confirmed by ultrasound. By this time, my body had completely regained its younger shape. I was born again."

"Why do you think Chi Lel helped you to recover while other types of qigong didn't?"

"It was the love I felt. The teachers cared about me and encouraged me when my spirits were low. Also, the Center provided me with an unshakable faith that I too, like many others, would be cured. The can-do attitude in the Center is contagious."

No wonder Teacher Zhou always has a smile and a caring attitude towards her students. Indeed, having been in their shoes before, she understands how important it is to show a little kindness to those who are in great need.

43. I Spat In My Wife's Face

While working on some electrical wiring in 1986, Teacher Yu was electrocuted. "I was dead for more than four hours, and when I woke up, the world had changed into a hazy place where I was always half-asleep. No longer able to work, I was idled at home at the age of thirty-one.

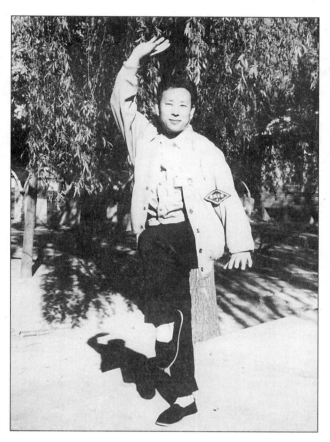

Yu Tian-Ming, 40, teacher

"Besides the fact that my head wasn't functioning normally, I also had many other ailments. Walking was difficult for me because my knees were stiff after surgeries. Eating was also a challenge as my throat hurt each time I swallowed food.

"Without knowing it, I expressed my sufferings through anger. My wife, understanding that my temper was due to my illness, was very patient with me. Once, when she peeled a grape and fed it to me, instead of appreciating her love I spat the grape out in her face. Every time I recall this incident, I still feel ashamed of my beastly act. Yet because of it, I am a better teacher, understanding what my students go through."

"So when did you begin your Chi Lel?"

"In May 1993 It was my sister's idea and she paid my expenses to come to the Center. Yet because of bad experiences during the Cultural Revolution, I was a deeply skeptical person. When I saw Lao-shi helping people to walk, talk, and see, I dismissed it as mass hysteria. When people talked about their miraculous recoveries, I thought they were either exaggerating or that their recoveries could have happened anywhere."

"When your own illnesses began to disappear, did you change your mind then?"

Teacher Yu surprised me by saying, "No."

"Why?"

"I don't know exactly, but somehow I didn't believe my recoveries were due to chi. Probably in my subconscious, I was suspicious of others who could have manipulated me like a fool. So I went home, knowing I had been cured, but nonetheless a doubter.

"When people found out that I had been in the Center, they asked me to teach them Chi Lel. Well it was no big deal for me to teach them in the park. One day someone asked me to emit chi to him in order to facilitate his healing, and when I did, he claimed that he was cured. I dismissed it as a student being polite. However, as I performed more Chi-Lel healings, people kept telling me the same thing.

"Without trying, I had become a well-known healer in my area. Then one day a relative came to me requesting that I perform a healing on him. But I refused because I am was not a doctor and I didn't want to bear any responsibility if he died. 'But the doctors have already sentenced me to death! Please help me,' he pleaded, with his family at his side.

"I finally agreed to try, but told his family not to blame me if he died, adding, 'I am treating a dead horse as if it were alive.' After a week of Chi-Lel treatment, the patient became more spirited and could sleep well. However, when he later reacted to chi by developing a high fever and having frequent bowel movements, I became worried. Immediately, I sent him to the Center, where he recovered a month later.

"After this event, I was totally convinced of the existence of chi and its power, and I have been an ardent supporter of Lao-shi ever since."

"What would you recommend to people who are skeptical about the effectiveness of Chi Lel?"

"Just do it first; chi will communicate to you later."

44. A Dead Man's Last Gamble

When Mr. Li told me that he only took medicine during the three years he had bladder cancer, I asked, "Didn't the doctors recommend surgery or chemotherapy?"

"No, although I was only fifty-eight at the time, they told me that I was too old for any of that.

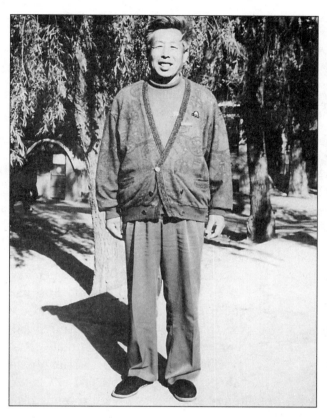

Li Cai, 61, student

Figuring doctors know best, I accepted my fate and watched my cancer grow bigger every day. Then in February of this year, doctors told my son that I had only three months to live. The news didn't surprise me because death was the logical conclusion of my incurable disease.

"My daughter, who lives in Qinhuangdao, asked me to visit her for the last time and do some sightseeing as well. In fact, she had prepared my 'longevity clothes' for me to bring home.

"While on the way to visit my daughter, I met a stranger on the train. He was very kind and asked me why I was having difficulty sitting down. After learning of my illness, he told me about Chi-Lel therapy at the Center in Qinhuangdao—right in my daughter's backyard.

"Getting off the train at Qinhuangdao, I was looking for a taxi instead of my daughter. With no time to waste, I wanted to go to the Center immediately. On our way to the Center, I asked my daughter why she didn't know about this place. She replied, 'I've heard of it, but have never paid much attention to it. If I am sick, I go to the hospital; after all, if Chi Lel is so effective, what are hospitals for?'

"However, my daughter didn't discourage me from going to the Center. By not doing so, she allowed me to indulge a dead man's last gamble in peace.

"Seeing so many people fighting their incurable diseases in the Center, I at last felt at home. Deep in my heart, I was determined to fight my illness until it died or I did."

"Why would you rather die here?"

"Chi Lel gave me a fighting chance to live. When I was doing Chi Lel, my body sweat, my legs shook, my hands were tired but my spirits were high. Summoning all my might, I was fighting back at my disease instead of waiting hopelessly at home and letting it eat me alive. Even if Chi Lel didn't work, I still felt the dignity of fighting gallantly instead of surrendering without a shot.

"So I practiced Chi Lel diligently day after day. After one month, I had regained some of my strength and could sleep and eat well. I continued to practice diligently and, with the help and caring of my teachers, I beat my cancer. Using ultrasound, the doctors couldn't find any trace of cancer in my bladder. My cancer was actually gone! When I broke the news to my family, they cried. I'm glad that they were happy tears."

This dead man had survived to tell his tale.

45. A Skeleton Soldier

In 1994, just before Mr. Shu was to become an army officer, his weight dropped from 154 to 99 pounds in only a few months. Subsequent examinations revealed that he had both a tumor growing above his stomach, and a 2x2 cm. lump in his lungs, which was possibly cancerous.

"When doctors suggested surgery to remove my tumors, I hesitated. How could I be a soldier without a strong body? Certainly my career would be over and probably also my life, for surgeries can be harbingers of worse yet to come.

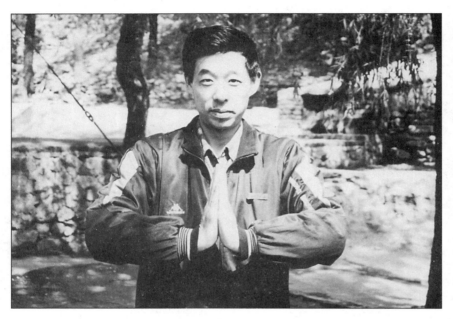

Shu Wei, 41, student

"I spent a couple of sleepless nights mulling over my options. In fact, the doctors hadn't given me any options at all—either I would undergo surgery or I wouldn't. If I didn't, my tumors would keep growing. 'How large is your body cavity?' my doctor would ask.

"Then one day while walking on the street with my head down, feeling hopeless, someone called my name, 'Shu Wei!' Looking up, I saw a stranger waving his hand. The man came over and asked, 'Don't you remember me? We shared the same hospital room last year.' Then it dawned on me that this was the same guy who had been dying in the hospital. 'Remember how we discussed the possibility of going to the Chi-Lel Center together while we were roommates?

I've just come back from there; it changed my life. Just look at me.' My old roommate turned around with much enthusiasm.

"Suddenly, I felt joy. If Chi Lel could help my friend, it certainly could help me too. So, after writing down the Center's address, I departed for there the next morning."

"Why did you decide so quickly that Chi Lel was for you?"

"There was no time to reach another conclusion. I didn't need further proof that Chi Lel could work because it had already worked for my friend, whose suffering I knew all too well. Besides, I am a very competitive person and have always believed that I can overcome any obstacle if given a chance to do something about it. Since I could take an active part in my own Chi-Lel therapy, I knew I could do it.

"Once at the Center, I was always the first to get up among the eight people in my room, usually at three or four o'clock in the morning; and the last one to sleep, often at eleven or twelve o'clock at night. In addition to our eight-hour-plus Chi-Lel routine, each day I did countless repetitions of Wall Squatting and massaged my abdomen whenever I had time.

"After two months in the Center, all my symptoms disappeared. Using the ultrasound, doctors couldn't find any trace of tumors inside my body. I was cured. Yet to keep up discipline, I still rise early and go to bed late. In this war against my illnesses I mustn't let up."

In the battle against his disease, Soldier Shu used neither guns nor knives; Chi Lel was his lethal weapon.

46. I Have Only One Bladder, Please Don't Cut It

"In April of 1991 I had surgery to remove my bladder cancer, and during the next three years, underwent chemotherapy and radiation treatments. Unfortunately, when the cancer didn't go away, the doctors told me they would have to remove my entire bladder.

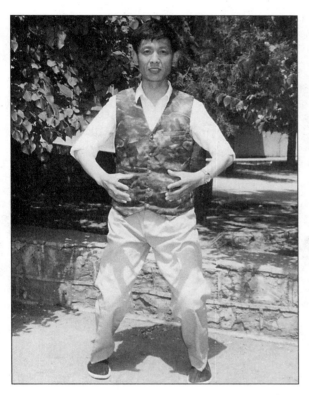

Xu Feng, 40, student

"However, even if they cut away my bladder, they couldn't guarantee that my cancer wouldn't reappear. After so much fruitless suffering, I had lost confidence in the ability of doctors to heal me. Besides, I have only one bladder and once it's gone, it can't be replaced. So I decided that if I was going to die, I would rather die with my bladder intact. Since I was still under doctors' care, I had to make up an excuse to get away from the hospital, telling the doctors I would be right back."

"So you escaped from the hospital?"

"Yes, I did, and I never went back. Soon a friend, whose uterine tumor had been cured in the Center, visited me and suggested that I learn Chi Lel. At first, I wasn't interested because I had studied other types of qigong before, with no effect. However, my friend persisted, describing many examples of people with different types of cancer who had been cured by practicing Chi Lel. Often she would say, 'Since you are preparing to die anyway, why not give Chi Lel a try?' Although her talks gave me much encouragement, I still would not allow myself to hope for the impossible.

"Finally, after having made all my burial arrangements, and with my wife accompanying me, I arrived at the Center last March. As soon as we got off the train, there were teachers from the Center welcoming us. Instead of treating me as a terminally ill patient, the teachers addressed me as "student." When one of the teachers told me that I was Lao-shi's guest and welcome, I was moved to tears.

"Reaching the Center, I felt very much at home. Seeing everyone in the Center working diligently, I got the message: If I wanted to live I must practice to death. So even in my feeble condition, I kept up with others. In addition, I began doing the Wall Squatting exercise. At first I was only able to do ten at a time, but eventually I could do fifty, and then one hundred. My condition improved daily.

"Then on April 26th, I was asked to undergo a chi treatment in connection with an ultrasound machine. I was happy to do it. With four teachers simultaneously emitting chi to me, my cancer disappeared in eleven seconds!"

"What were you thinking while the teachers were emitting chi to you?"

"Glory to our country! I wanted my cancer to go away so that the whole world could see it. At the time a German TV station was videotaping the procedure.

"Besides healing my cancer, Chi Lel also cured my wife of the dizziness and shaky legs that she'd had since a motorcycle accident. We are one happy couple now."

47. My Wife, Please Don't Let Our Friends Laugh at Us

Ms. Liu, a mother of two young children, was worried when she was hospitalized for diabetes, accompanied by bad vision, no appetite, high blood pressure, chest pain, and a rapid heart rate. Although she was still feeling sick, the doctors sent her home, telling her she needed plenty of rest.

"They said, 'don't worry about anything, don't do vigorous exercises, and of course don't forget to take your medicine.' How could I not worry? How would I take care of my children if I continued to be sick like this? Would I be sitting at home doing nothing for the rest of my life? But what could I do? I had heard that diabetes is a disease that accompanies people to their graves.

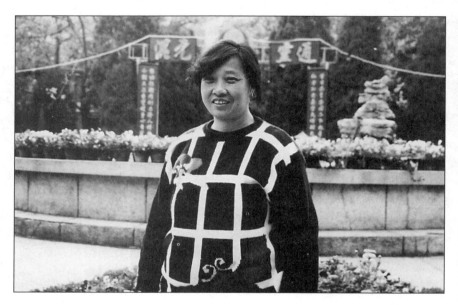

Liu Feng-Yun, 42, student

"Then one day a neighbor told me that many people with diabetes had been cured at the Chi-Lel Center. Upon hearing such a good news, I immediately told my husband about it, expecting him to share my excitement.

"'Chi Lel?' my husband snorted with contempt, 'Don't you know our neighbor? She's a liar. If there were such a way to treat diabetes, why haven't the doctors told us? I know that you're anxious to get well, but my wife, please don't let our friends laugh at us.' After listening to my husband's 'sensible' talk, I abandoned the idea of going to the Center.

"However, my condition continued to deteriorate, reaching a point where I couldn't even go down a flight of stairs. Now my husband began to feel the effect of my illness as he had to take care of the whole household. So when our neighbor mentioned the Center again, my husband's attitude had changed and he asked me to try it.

"My husband escorted me to the Center three months ago. In the Center, my illnesses didn't frighten me anymore because I witnessed many people with even worse diseases being cured. With a belief that I could heal myself, I practiced Chi Lel assiduously for eight hours or more a day. By the end of the first month, my heartbeat had slowed down, my chest pain had disappeared and the sugar levels in my blood and urine had decreased. By the end of the second month, my heart had returned to normal and my diabetes was gone. I felt energetic and could eat and drink."

"What did you think about when you were practicing Chi Lel?"

"I would imagine my entire body becoming permeable to chi while affirming repeatedly to myself that I was a healthy person."

"In other words, you were willing to open yourself up for life energy, chi, to enter your body?"

"Yes, when I opened up to the universal energy, my illnesses disappeared and I returned to my natural state."

Indeed, Ms. Liu had returned to a state of happiness and well being.

48. A Young Principal Couldn't Make It to the Bathroom

Mr. Peng, a vice principal of a prestigious high school in Nanking, became seriously ill in February of 1994.

"One morning I woke up to find myself unable to move. I was sent to a hospital immediately and doctors told me that the muscles in my body were shrinking and becoming brittle. They called my illness a severe case of polymyositis. Four months later, before they sent me home, they advised me, 'Be very careful at home, please don't move much.'

"At home, I spent most of my time in the bed, with my medications making me fat."

"Could you do any exercise?"

"No, my muscles seemed to get worse the more I moved them. I even needed my wife's help to go to the bathroom. What was I looking forward to? One of our school's teachers who had a similar disease died within a year after his being diagnosed—was it my turn next?"

"So you turned to Chi Lel?"

"Yes and no, my first experience with Chi Lel wasn't a positive one. When a Chi-Lel practitioner who is a college professor and a friend of mine emitted chi to me, my muscles swelled up even more. Unaware that my muscles were responding to chi, I was afraid to do any more Chi Lel. However, my friend taught me the simple exercise La Chi, of opening and closing my hands, and left me with a Chi-Lel book.

"As I was lying in bed, I started to read the Chi-Lel book. The more I read, the more the book made sense. I began to open and close my hands eight to nine hours a day, continuously wishing that chi would come to me. At first I only lay in my bed, then gradually I moved to a chair to do the movements, and later to a standing position. Meanwhile, I learned from the book to do other Chi-Lel movements as well.

"After three weeks, I could walk short distances and had stopped taking the fattening drugs. I no longer needed assistance in my daily life.

Peng Jian-Guo, 42, student

"When the Center reopened March 1st after being closed for the winter, my wife accompanied me there. Like a bird out of its cage, I felt so free and happy in the Center, and, after just two months of intensive Chi Lel, I could both jump and run."

To prove his abilities, the school principal jumped up and down like a schoolchild at recess.

"Will you teach Chi Lel to your students?"

"Yes indeed, to anyone who will listen. But it won't be easy."

"What do you mean? Aren't your a good advertisement for Chi Lel?"

"True, but chi is an empty concept if one doesn't feel it. In order to feel chi and get its benefits, one must concentrate while practicing Chi Lel. How do you motivate people to concentrate on doing something every day for a long period of time? It's not easy. It took a life-threatening disease for me to do so."

What about those people who are motivated, but don't know about Chi Lel? I wonder if Chi Lel could have saved the life of principal Peng's diseased colleague?

49. My Aunt Saved Me

Ms. Wang became sick when she was thirty-eight years old. She had low blood pressure, and a slow heart rate of forty beats per minute. Because her heart wasn't supplying enough oxygen to her brain, she was dizzy most of the time and tended to faint easily. In addition, she couldn't squat down or bear the touch of cold water because of arthritis in her joints. In short, her life was miserable.

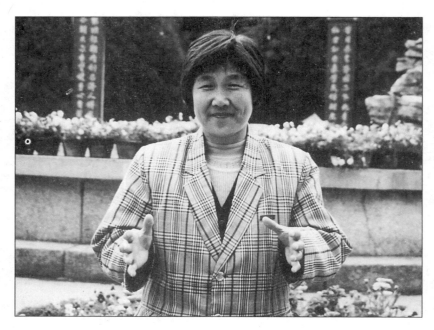

Wang Rui-Chin, 53, student

"I was angry at myself and the world. Why me? I would lay awake at night feeling frustrated. There was nothing I could do to alleviate my pain except to take more and more drugs."

"Nothing you could do? With so many people exercising in the parks, why didn't you join them?"

"It might seem strange to you, but I was trapped in my own small world, thinking my illnesses were unique to me. When the doctors told me that I should have plenty of rest and take medicine on a regular basis, I followed their advice faithfully. Exercising, even gently, would rob me of my resting time—I wanted to live!"

"So why did you change your mind and seek an alternative way of healing yourself after fifteen years of taking medication?"

"My aunt opened my mind. When she was first diagnosed with liver cancer, I felt sorry for her. But then only a few months later, I was surprised to see my aunt. Instead of a skeleton lying in a hospital bed as I had last seen her, she was a healthy, spirited and much younger looking person. Her secret? Chi Lel. 'Niece, why don't you learn a self-healing art? You have suffered enough,' she said, embracing me.

"Witnessing my aunt's recovery made my illnesses not seem so untouchable anymore. So, in my uncle's company, I came to the Center last month. Once at the Center, I felt as though I belonged here. All eyes seemed to tell me that they understood. In fact, many of us who had once floundered helplessly on the sea now were being saved by this ship.

"With hope and newfound faith, I began to do the opposite of standard doctors' advice: 'get plenty of rest.' Pampering my illnesses no more, I did Chi Lel until I was exhausted and then continued. No more drugs for me! I would rather die here with dignity than die slowly at home.

"With such determination, I made great progress in a short time. After a month, my blood pressure increased to 80/120 and an EKG showed a normally functioning heart. Not only are there are no more swellings in my joints, but I can eat and sleep well. I feel great!"

Ms. Wang smiled broadly. For her, life was more precious now than ever. Having once lost her health, she had found it again!

50. Welcome Home

"I had liver cancer surgery last April, but unfortunately, three months later, the cancer spread to my lungs. My whole family cried as the doctor predicted that I would be dead in about two months.

"Luckily, my neighbor was a Chi-Lel teacher and he taught me the art of self-healing. After practicing Chi Lel, my cancer was stabilized. Then on the first day of March this year, I was able to travel to the Center.

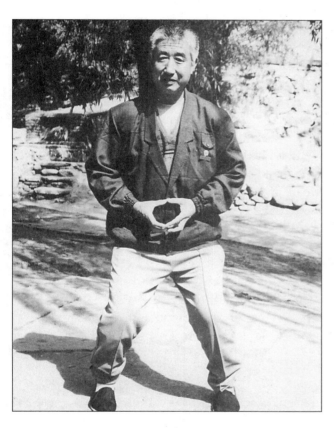

Li Chong-Cheng, 50, student

"I remember vividly the moment I stepped out of the railway station and saw many teachers standing in line to welcome me. People were coming from all parts of the country, some in wheelchairs, some walking on crutches, some like myself being helped by family members, and many others, young and old, carrying suitcases of clothes and daily necessities, all coming to the Center with a dream—to be free of their illnesses.

"The teachers had arranged for buses to bring us to the Center. Once we were on the bus, our teacher said, 'Welcome, students, you must be tired after such a long journey. With all our hearts, we welcome you to the Chi-Lel Center. From now on you are Lao-shi's guests and the Center is your home. Welcome home!'

"Our teacher said this with such sincerity that many of us were moved to tears. Indeed, many of the people on this bus had, like myself, reached a deadend after being turned away from hospitals as incurable. We now regarded the Center as our last hope. Yes, we had finally come home—to live or to die, without regret.

"With such a warm reception at the station, my body began to heal from the very beginning. I followed my teacher's instructions closely and practiced Chi Lel harder than anyone else. Deep into the night, I often practiced alone while others slept. After two months, my cancer was gone and I had gained almost twenty pounds."

"Can you explain how you achieved this incredible recovery?"

"While doing the Three Centers Merge Standing Method, I would imagine my body becoming empty, without ever thinking of my illness. Sometimes I would even fall asleep while standing."

"Tell me, how could you forget an illness which loomed over you as a shadow of death, ready to snatch you any time? Was it not a killing disease?"

"Yes, it was a killing disease all right and I have a doctor's diagnosis to prove it; nonetheless, I could just forget it while doing Chi Lel. I can't explain how my mind worked. Maybe I was a good student, because when my teacher told me to empty my mind and not to be preoccupied with my illness, I just listened and did what I was told."

Being an obedient student, Mr. Li lived to tell his tale.

51. A Long March

Manager Liu is a friendly, easygoing person who has the important post of overseeing hundreds of office personnel in the Center. One day while we were having lunch together, he volunteered to talk about his experience.

"I come from a military background. Back in 1978, I was diagnosed with a severe case of diabetes. After spending months in the hospital, I returned home as a 'medicine bag,' relying totally on medication to survive. Within a year, I became too weak to function on my job, and so, at the age of forty-two, in the prime of my life, I was forced into early retirement."

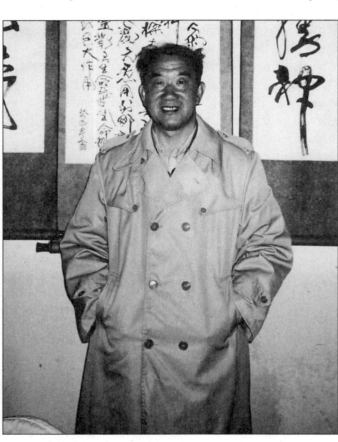

Liu Chang-Ting, 58, office manager

"Did you take up Chi Lel immediately?"

"No. At the time, Chi Lel was not known to the general public because China was just opening up after the fall of the Gang of Four. It was not until 1987 that I began learning Chi Lel.

"Even with Chi Lel, I battled my illness for two years before subduing it. During this two-year period, my blood sugar level often fluctuated."

"What went through your mind during your long journey?"

"Each time I practiced Chi Lel, I treated it as a step in my Long March to final victory. Even after my full recovery in 1989, I have never let up in my practice. Chi Lel is as much a part of my life as eating and sleeping."

"Manager Liu, I have interviewed many students who recovered from their illnesses in only a month or two. Why did it take you two years to overcome yours?"

"Each individual takes a different route to recovery. Here at the Center, students can recover faster because of the healing atmosphere."

"What do you mean?"

"Among many other factors, living examples like myself are very important for students to identify with in order to build up confidence. If students have faith in Chi Lel, they already have half their battle won. At the Center, there are hundreds if not thousands of incredible healing stories for students to hear and see. That's why people recover faster here."

"Can Americans duplicate these results?"

"Chi is universal. You should bring back our stories to America and let people know that we exist. Of course, we welcome American friends to visit us anytime to share our experience."

I thanked Manager Liu and promised that I would be back soon with some foreign friends.

52. Like Floating On Air

After discovering she had ovarian cancer in September 1994, Ms. Sun followed the advice of her doctor to have surgery, followed by five chemotherapy sessions. Unfortunately, the cancer reappeared seven months later and the doctor suggested another surgery.

"Surgery again? Will it end up being just as fruitless as the first one? Just when I was hesitating to have another operation, a friend told me about Chi Lel. But I didn't have faith in Chi Lel either."

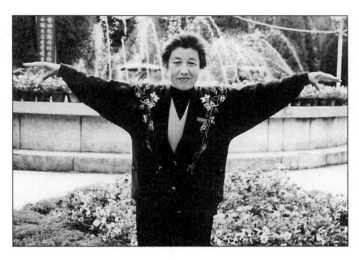

Sun Jin-Yun, 52, student

"Why not?"

"Being a government official, I'm not supposed to believe superstitious things. Because people can't see or touch chi, chi therapy is considered as unscientific. So when others would claim, without proof, that they could see or feel chi, I was suspicious of their motives."

"Then what changed your mind?"

"My attitude changed when my friend said, 'Even if Chi Lel doesn't heal you, it won't kill you.' In fact, I was afraid of death at the time.

"Strangely, once I decided to put my life in the hands of Chi Lel, I felt relieved—as if I had given up on my old life in order for a new one to sprout within me.

"With new hope, I was escorted by my family to the Center a few weeks ago. My body reacted instantly to the healing energy here. Indeed, I felt light, as if floating on air. In a few days, the doctors told me that my cancer had disappeared. What a good piece of news!"

"What do you think was the reason that you were able to just 'absorb' the life energy and get well so soon?"

"I'm not sure. Maybe I was willing to let go of my old self and let in a new one. Or maybe my chi is very compatible with the healing chi in the Center. For whatever reason, I was cured. But I am not letting down my guard. I practice Chi Lel diligently every day like everybody else in the Center and I have no intention of slowing down."

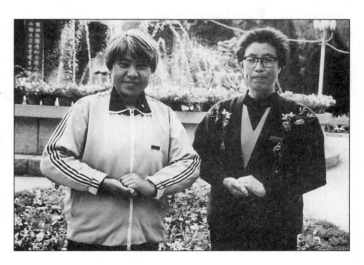

Sun Jin-Yun and Guo Ya-Chin

When I asked Ms. Sun if she had told her friend about the good news, she suddenly pointed to someone who just happened to be passing by: "That's my friend. You should interview her."

At first her friend was taken aback by someone from America wanting to interview her. But, after learning my intentions, she was happy to tell me about her life (see next interview).

53. A Woman Warrior

Underneath her soft, gentle voice, Ms. Guo had tremendous strength of body and mind. This was clear as her story unfolded.

"Two years ago, I declared war on my illness. Now, even though I have won a battle, I continue to fight my enemies to the death."

"What battle have you won?"

"I have beaten cancer. Back in February 1993, I had surgery to remove my cancer. But the cancer reappeared, and while still undergoing chemotherapy, spread to my lymph nodes. I was done for—at least that's what the doctors said.

"Just when I thought my life had reached a dead end, my husband, a college professor, learned about Chi Lel from a colleague and encouraged me to try it."

"Were you surprised when your scholarly husband asked you to learn Chi Lel?"

"No, my husband has an open mind, and since I had tried everything that modern hospitals have to offer without results, it was time to search out other alternatives.

"Before I went to the Center, I read one of Laoshi's books which emphasized that if one could concentrate and work very hard on practicing Chi Lel, one could overcome all illnesses. This aroused a warrior attitude within me to fight my cancer until either I died or it disappeared."

"How did you fight?"

"I got up earlier and went to bed later than anybody else in the Center and practiced Chi Lel whenever awake. By accepting the fact that my survival depended on my personal efforts, I felt my destiny was in my own hands. So if I died, I would die in glory as a gallant fighter; and if I lived, my life would become more precious. Since all my time was spent in practicing Chi Lel, I had no time to worry about my illness. By forgetting my disease, I was able to concentrate on collecting life energy into my body. With such a fighting spirit, I beat my cancer within three months."

Guo Ya-Chin, 51, student

"It was two years ago that your cancer was cured. Why are you here now?"

"I come back to the Center every year to rekindle my fighting spirit. Even though I have won a battle, I must keep a vigilant eye on different diseases that might pop up. I figure in the long run I will spend less time practicing Chi Lel every day than I would waste being sick."

"Do you think people have the discipline to follow a daily Chi-Lel routine?"

"Once people are aware of Chi Lel's curative and preventive functions, they will naturally do it daily, in much the same way as they brush their teeth."

54. That's My Toe

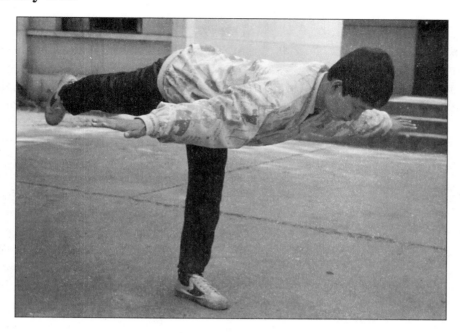

Zhang Hung-Sun, 20, instructor trainee

With my pen and notebook ready, I looked directly at Mr. Zhang, expecting him to tell me a story of his struggle for life. I was surprised when he pointed to his foot and said, "It was my toe."

"What was wrong with your toe?"

"I cut my left foot in an accident six years ago. When the wound healed I found my big toe had no feeling, no response to cold or heat or any outside stimulation. The doctors told me that the nerves in my toe were damaged and that I should simply learn to live with a numb toe."

"So you have decided to take up Chi Lel in order to deal with the situation?"

"No, I came to the Center to learn Chi Lel for strengthening my body. I never thought of my toe because I had already been living without it for six years.

"Then after two months of Chi Lel, somehow the nerves in my left toe re-established themselves with my brain. As I began to again have feeling in my toe, I realized how much I had missed it. I am quite happy that my toe has finally awakened from a six- year-sleep!"

"Well, that's very interesting, Mr. Zhang. But it is only a toe."

"Yes, sir, *but it's my toe that we are talking about*! Besides, how often have you heard of nerves being regenerated?"

"Let me ask you, Mr. Zhang, if it had been one of your feet instead of your toes, could its nerves have been regenerated by practicing Chi Lel?"

"If chi works on a toe, it will surely work on other parts of the body as well. In the world of chi, nothing is impossible."

"What do you want to do after graduation?"

"I want to become a Chi-Lel teacher."

With such unshaken believe in chi, Mr. Zhang is bound to become an excellent healer.

55. Hey, What's Wrong With You?

Although Ms. Wang talked in an unfamiliar dialect, I had no trouble understanding her animated gestures.

"For the past fourteen years, I walked with my left shoulder higher than my right shoulder and I couldn't bend my body. I had constant back pain. I tried both Western and Chinese medicines and acupuncture, but nothing seemed to help. With my husband's encouragement, my daughter and I came to the Center last month.

"After a long trip on the train, I was very tired. While waiting in line to register for the class, I felt someone pat me on my left shoulder, saying, 'Hey, what's wrong with you?' As though awakening from a dream, I responded by straightening my body! Then I saw a Chi-Lel teacher smiling. My body has remained straight ever since." As she spoke, Ms. Wang stood up to re-enact the scene.

"Since you were healed on your very first day here, did you want to go home right away?"

"Are you kidding?" a young woman next to her interrupted. "My mother plunged right into Chi-Lel practice. I asked her to slow down when I saw her sweating profusely in the sun, but she scolded me for disturbing her."

"Are you here to take care of your mother?"

"Only in part," she replied with a big grin. "I had diabetes before I came here. My blood sugar level was 8.1 and in my urine the sugar was 4.0. But the doctors now tell me they are normal, and I am one happy woman."

Indeed, two miracles occurred in one family.

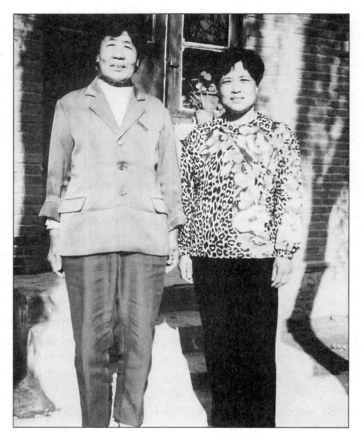

Wang Bao-Ming(l), 67, student
Zhang Ming-Hua(r), 42, student

56. She Sang After Fifty Years

Ms. Chin had been depressed for the last fifty years and had not sung since she was twenty-two years old.

"I was branded as a 'bad element' by the government and suffered tremendously during every revolution. At first, I pretended to be sad and crazy so that people would leave me alone. Later it became reality. I would never smile or sing and usually acted a little nutty. During those years I also developed nephritis and a peptic ulcer. So, mentally I was locked in my own prison and physically I was dependent on drugs.

"Just as I was about to write off my life as an unhappy one, someone told me about the Center. So I came here, hoping to cure my kidney and intestinal diseases."

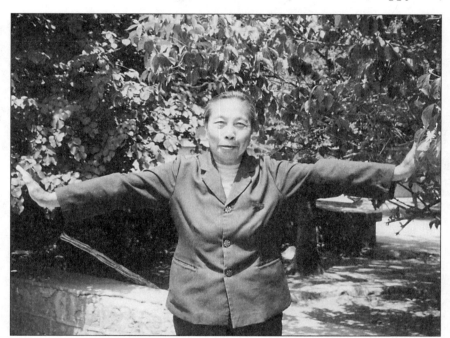

Chin Jing-Ru, 72, student

"At your age, could you follow the Center's intensive training schedule?"

"I adapted to the routine quickly. In the Center, I felt ten years younger because of my roommates' encouragement. The eight of us, living under one roof, quickly became good friends. I even began to sing and laugh. How exonerated I felt when I heard myself singing and caught myself laughing after fifty years! My depression seemed to dissipate with each song and laugh.

"Along with my depression, my kidneys and intestines also were healed. One time I vomited a lot of black stuff, but this was a sign of healing. Now my body has rejuvenated itself and I hope to live to be a hundred."

As I was concluding the interview with Ms. Chin and her roommates, I requested that they sing their Center's song so that I could hear Ms. Chin's singing. They huddled together and sang the following:

"We're from every corner of the world
With one ideal—Discover the mystery of life, free ourselves
Come to the Zhineng Gong school
Diligently practice; perfect body and mind
Harmonious, happy, natural, polite
Intelligence uncommon; high moral standards
Free ourselves; free ourselves
Let's run toward utopia; run toward utopia
On a broad way."

They sang with such love and sincerity that I was moved to tears.

57. I Had Prepared My Own Funeral Clothes

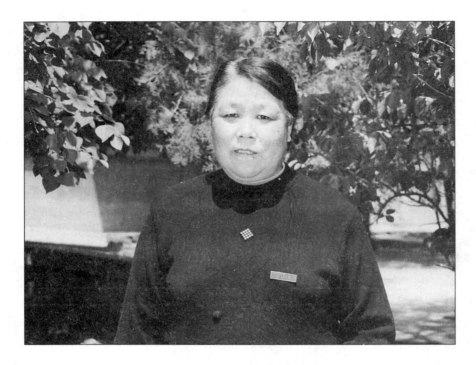

Wen Bao-Zhen, 59, student

Ms. Wen had high blood pressure for many years. Last year she was operated on for a cerebral hemorrhage, and, after the surgery, was unable to walk. The doctors were pessimistic about her recovery.

"After listening to my doctors, I understood my chance of survival was slim. So I prepared my funeral clothes and waited in bed for my final exit.

"Then someone told me about the Center. At first, I didn't want to go because I was too weak to travel by myself. If I was going to die anyway, why make more trouble for my family? But my children insisted that I should try.

"So with my son carrying me on his back and my daughter holding me, I came to the Center two months ago. Strangely, during my first day in the Center, I could stand up and walk a few steps. Following my teacher's instructions, I was able to practice Chi Lel with others.

"After shaking hands with Lao-shi, I developed a high fever. My teacher and classmates came to emit chi to me, encouraging me to hang on to life."

"Did you call for a doctor?"

"What doctor? I was happy to know my body was reacting to chi, dissipating my illness in the form of a fever. Since then my blood pressure has returned to normal and I am no longer taking any medication."

"What are you going to do with your funeral clothes?"

"Well, I've never thought about it. What can I do with my funeral clothes? They won't be new if I wait until I can use them; it wouldn't be polite to give them to others. I'm in a dilemma. Any suggestions?"

"Why don't you ask your doctor?"

Ms. Wen laughed heartily, "True, very true."

58. I Don't Want to Leave

"Five months?" I asked in surprise when Ms. Yu told me that she had spent five months in the Center. "Yes, and I don't want to leave."

"What illness did you have?"

"I developed coronary disease when I was forty-seven. My illness put a halt to any social activities because my heart would race whenever I got excited. My career was finished because I could no longer compete in my job without putting my life in jeopardy. Then a friend told me about Chi Lel and its Center. So I came here to give it a try.

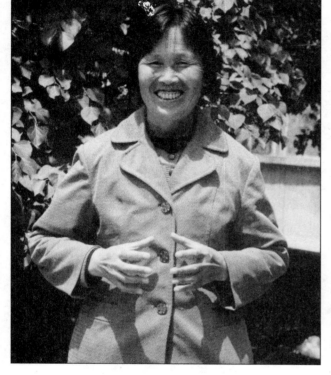

Yu Shu-Jun, 52, student

"When I first arrived, I was afraid to do any bending movements because I thought they might be harmful to my heart. But when I saw so many people with severe heart problems doing the movements, I finally believed my teacher when she said that all the Chi-Lel movements had been thoroughly tested by millions of people. With faith, I began to follow everything done in the Center and recovered in a couple of months. I am no longer taking any medicine and an EKG has shown my heart to be normal.

"I remember when I was hospitalized for my illness a few years ago, I couldn't wait to get out the hospital. But here in the Center, I didn't want to leave because I enjoyed the company of my roommates. In the beginning, we were strangers coming from different parts of China, now we are friends helping each other. Once, when I was too weak to do my laundry, my roommates competed to help me. Now that I am cured, I am competing to help those roommates who are still in need."

"You are not worried about money?"

"No, the amount of money I have spent here is very little compared with regular hospitals. Six hundred yuans is enough for one month's expenses, including tuition, room, and board. The Center is here to serve us, not to earn money from us. We are all grateful to Lao-shi."

"How much do you have to pay for tuition and your room?"

"I, like all other students, pay 100 yuan tuition fee each month and 6 yuan per bed per night. The fee is higher for those rooms with less people. I prefer the size of eight."

"Don't you want privacy?"

"Being sick is a very lonesome thing. With more people, you don't have much quiet time to dwell on illnesses; and, with the encouragement and love of roommates, you can recover faster. Besides, living alone is more expensive."

"How long will you stay at the Center?"

"A month or two. I guess the banquet has to end some time, but until then I am enjoying every minute of it."

Indeed, the Center is not only a place for the sick, it is also an oasis for the cured and the healthy. Its founder, Lao-shi, deserves our utmost respect.

59. This Doctor Quit Her Job As a Medicine Dispenser

Dr. Zhang is one of twenty-six doctors trained in Western medicine who work at the Center. Out of respect, people address her as Teacher Zhang instead of Dr. Zhang. In the Center, students pay more attention to teachers than doctors.

"Even though in my hometown I was the chief internist of a major hospital, I was unable to cure my own coronary disease, chronic bronchitis, and rheumatoid arthritis. Since I worked in a hospital, I could freely take all the drugs I needed. In 1988, I was involuntarily retired.

"With nothing to do after retirement, I went to the parks to learn some exercises. I learned many types of qigong. However, I decided to give up all other forms of exercise and practice Chi Lel exclusively."

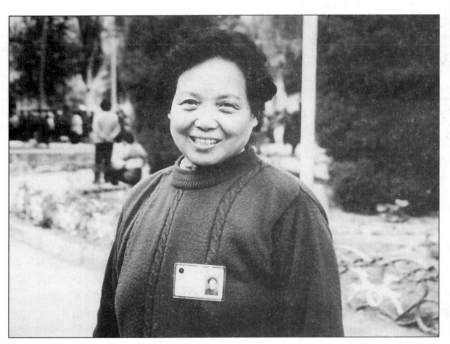

Zhang Chang-Rong, 64, M.D.

"What prompted you to make that decision?"

"Two reasons. First, Chi Lel is more scientific, it doesn't have any overtones of superstition. Second, Chi Lel has a theoretical foundation, based on the writings by Lao-shi. As a scientist myself, I enjoy practicing something that is theoretically sound and believable.

"Can't you practice more than one qigong at a time?"

"I didn't have much time. Besides, it is better to stick with one and get its benefits than practice all and end up with nothing. Just as if someone wants to be good at volleyball, one must spend time practicing volleyball not basketball and vice versa. Even though both sports use a ball as an object, the way of playing is different.

"Once my mind was made up, I practiced Chi Lel with all my heart. Eventually, all my illnesses had left me and I didn't need to take any medication anymore. I became so energetic that I wanted to go back to work."

"Did you go back to your hospital?"

"I had thought about it, but decided not to go back because I would return just as before, no more than a medicine dispenser. If I am not taking medicine anymore, how could I advise my patients to take them without reservation? Fortunately, the Center needed doctors and I came here two years ago."

"Tell me, Doctor, do people die here?"

"Yes, like in any big hospital, patients do die. Because many patients come to the Center in advanced stages of disease, some do eventually succumb to their illnesses. But there is a big difference between the Center and other hospitals—in the Center, patients die with dignity, free of pain. And the family members of those who die are very grateful to the teachers for treating their loved ones kindly and giving them hope up to the last minute of their lives so that they could rest in peace, instead of fear."

Ultimately, everyone has to die. But how much better to die peacefully and with dignity, instead of being connected to tubes and taking painkillers.

60. An S-Shaped Creature Transformed Into a Beautiful Girl

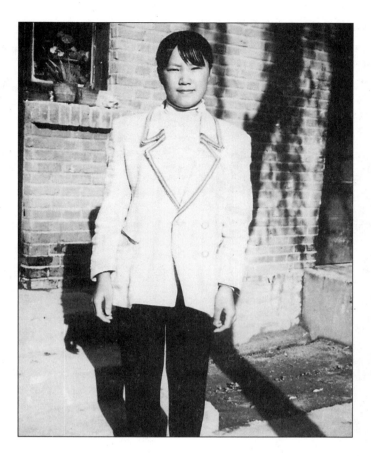

Xu Wei-Dong, 18, student

The next person I interviewed was a beautiful girl with a pair of sparkling eyes. Unlike most girls her age who enjoyed a normal life, she had gone through what she described as hell.

"Five years ago I developed the bad habit of bending my body to one side while carrying my schoolbag, and gradually my spine became crooked. My mother brought me to various doctors but none could help me. Finally, my body became S-shaped, with my head permanently bending to one side. I couldn't sleep at night because in every position I laid my body weight would press against my internal organs, making breathing difficult and very painful. As my condition worsened, doctors predicted that I would eventually die a painful death.

"Then one of our relatives heard of the Center and told us about it. My mother brought me here last month and a miracle happened on the first day. After my teacher emitted chi to me, my head moved to the center! For the first time in many years I could sleep without pain.

"My teacher told me that I must gather my own chi to heal myself completely. So I have been practicing Chi Lel more than eight hours a day. Now my body has returned to a normal shape."

"Do you have a picture of yourself with a S-shaped body?" As she shook her head uneasily, it dawned on me that most people pose for pictures when they are happy not when they are sad, let alone deformed.

61. An Old Martial Arts Champion

For a month, I shared a dinner table with this inspiring martial artist, who took first place in broadsword in 1933, during the Fifth National Martial Arts Competition. "We used real weapons. But later the competition was banned because of too many injuries."

In later years, Master Zhao was plagued with asthma, high blood pressure, heart disease, and body deformation. His expertise in martial arts was of no use in fighting these new enemies. So he turned to Chi Lel in 1988 for help, and, after two years, regained his health.

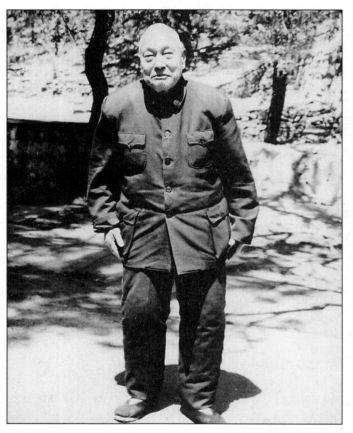

Zhao Chun-Sing, 83, student

"When I was cured of my heart condition and asthma, I wrote a thank-you letter to Lao-shi. In my letter I mentioned that I was an old champion and wished that I had used chi for health earlier in my life. Unexpectedly Lao-shi replied to my letter, inviting me to live at the Center free of charge. I am an old horse which has now found a green pasture. I bow to Lao-shi."

Everyday, Master Zhao would stand in the front row of his class, practicing Chi Lel just as seriously as the young. He also showed me neatly written notes on Chi Lel, which demonstrated his diligent reading on Chi-Lel theory.

During mealtime, I sometimes asked him, "Master Zhao, how was your day?" His answer was always the same, "Today the chi is plentiful. I feel very good."

Chi is life energy. With plenty of life energy, one can lead a long life. "Master Zhao, do you want to live to be a hundred?"

"One day at a time, young man. One day at a time."

At the age of eighty-three, Master Zhao still follows the Center's vigorous training schedule. He is an inspiration to people of all ages.

62. A Sportsman's Nightmare

Mr. Yu was studying to be a doctor when he was injured five years ago during a soccer game. Several back vertebrae and a pelvic joint were severely dislocated. For twelve days and nights, the future doctor leaned on a table, unable to either stand up or lay down. "What a nightmare! The slightest movement would cause a knifelike pain in my back—I couldn't even cry. It was a horrible experience.

"After that trauma, my body was never the same again. Even my memory started to slip, causing my studies to suffer. Where before the accident I was well ahead of the other students, after I lost my memory I could barely keep up with my medical school work. My height even shrank a few inches because I couldn't stand up straight anymore. My situation didn't improve even after I graduated from medical college."

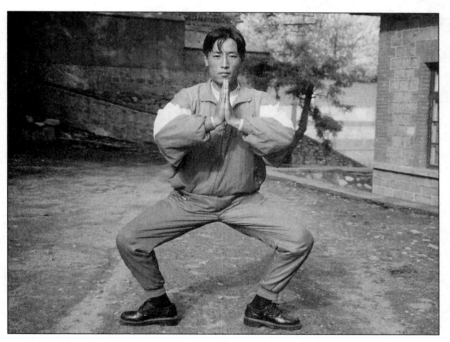

Yu Xian-Jun, M.D., 25, student

"What suggestions did your doctors give you about your situation?"

"What else? Surgery."

"Why didn't you take your colleagues' advice?"

"Are you kidding? As a doctor, I understood that once a back is cut open, there are so many delicate nerves inside that part of the body that a slight mistake can lead to permanent damage. Besides, the success rate of such operations is very low. That's why I chose to bear the pain rather than to risk an operation."

"Who told you about Chi Lel?"

"My college professor. When I heard the news, I was as happy and free as a fish finding water. For one thing, I trusted my professor. He is someone who won't believe anything unless he has closely examined it for himself. For another, being a sportsman, I liked what Chi Lel had to offer—exercises to heal oneself.

"So when I came to the Center last month and found what I had expected—work, work, and more work—I loved it! The teachers told us that if you could stand up to exercise, you should stand up; if you can only sit up, you should sit up; if you can only move while lying down, you should do the exercises in bed. In other words, unless you are dead, everyone here is expected to do Chi Lel.

"With that mentality, I met the challenge by doing Wall Squatting daily. The more pain I felt the more I moved. Against my enemy, there was no retreat. Through this process, my back straightened and my joints were brought back to their proper positions."

"So what will you tell your patients when you get back to your hospital, Dr. Yu?"

"I'm not sure if I want to go back. I hope to stay here."

63. A New Tooth Grew in an Old Mouth

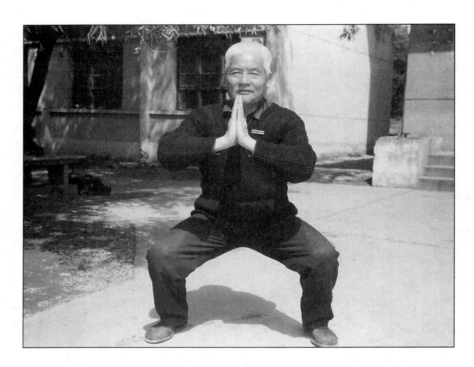

Zhang Yan-Zhao, 66, instructor trainee

Even before he reached the age of sixty, most of Mr. Zhang's teeth were gone. Besides being toothless, he also relied on crutches because of severe leg and back pains. In addition, he had had itchy urticaria all his life.

"My wife and I joined a Chi-Lel group in the park in July of 1991. At first, I felt a lot of pain because I was actually exercising my joints instead of avoiding their use in an effort to prevent pain. Gradually the pain became less and less because chi was lubricating my joints. A new life began to sprout out of my dead bones. Also, my skin disease disappeared as I continued to practice Chi Lel.

"My wife's high blood pressure was also cured by doing Chi Lel every day. We haven't felt this healthy since we were young. One day, I was surprised to find a new tooth growing in my gums!"

Mr. Zhang opened his mouth and showed a baby tooth to me. "It's a miracle. If even a tooth can grow back, it's no wonder I feel so good after practicing Chi Lel. I figure that the rest of my internal organs must have rejuvenated themselves like my tooth has done. And on my head, black hairs have started coming back."

Mr. Zhang proudly showed me a few shreds of black among his all gray hair. I imagine he was as surprised as someone else suddenly finding a few shreds of gray in their otherwise perfectly youthful hair. Of course, for Mr. Zhang it was a happy surprise.

"Mr. Zhang, have you heard stories that some masters live to be hundreds of years old?"

"Yes, I have and now I believe it is possible after all."

In fact, Lao-shi has plans to build a Chi-Lel City which will house many centenarians. Mr. Zhang will likely be among them.

64. Entering the Back Door to Recovery

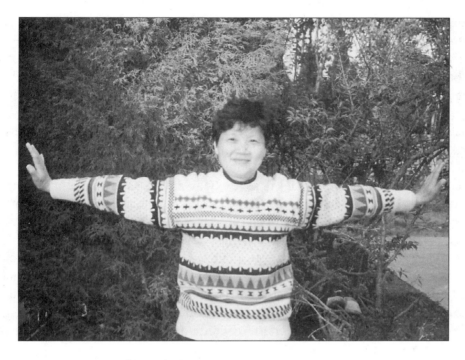

Chen Ai-Kun, 56, instructor trainee

With her smooth skin and fair complexion, Ms. Chen looked much younger than her age. Speaking in a soft voice, she described her heroic struggle against disease.

"As long as I can remember I have been fighting diseases. Besides suffering from diabetes and kidney disease, I had bladder stones in 1960, and a liver tumor in 1963. Just when I thought I'd had enough of surgeries, my thyroid gland became cancerous and required an operation in 1977. But the cancer didn't go away after this surgery and, a few years later, I underwent a second operation."

"So this time the cancer left for good?"

"That's what I thought at the time, but unfortunately, the cancer reappeared three years later. The doctors were now afraid to operate on me anymore and my cancer continued to grow as nothing was done about it for another three years. Finally, another hospital suggested that I undergo a third operation."

"Did you follow this advice?"

"It was very tempting because someone was at least trying to take care of the cancer instead of letting it eat me alive. But the doctors weren't sure if another surgery would help because it was likely that the cancer had spread to my bones. I couldn't move my left hand at all and my right hand only to chest level. I couldn't lay down to sleep because my back hurt and gradually, I lost my speech too. Finally, the doctors predicted that I had only two months to live."

"Did you cry upon hearing such dreadful news?"

"No."

"Why not?"

"I had no more tears to shed."

"So you had given up?"

"Not quite. I was used to bad news. So when my sister, who was practicing medicine in Beijing, invited me to live with her for my final days, I jumped at the chance. Once in Beijing, I saw hundreds of people practicing Chi Lel and became curious to learn it."

"How could you do Chi Lel if you couldn't even move your hands?"

"That's what I wondered at first. But my teacher told me that I should move as much as I could with my body and use my mind to gather life energy from the universe. I believed him and practiced diligently. Gradually, I regained my speech and could take care of myself."

"So you recovered completely and lived happily ever after?"

"Not yet. After a year's practice, I decided that I was well enough to go to the Center for further training. However, I was turned away by the Center."

"Are you kidding? I've been told that the Center is a place of mercy."

"Yes, but it has a rule that anyone who is severely ill should have an accompanying family member as a caretaker. They told me that the Center was a self-help place and students need to help themselves to get meals, take baths, and so on."

"Did you then go home and bring your sister with you?"

"No, I felt I had already burdened my sister too much. Fortunately my Chi-Lel teacher, who just happened to be at the Center, persuaded the registrar to admit me through the back door.

"But when I told my teacher that I wanted to register as an instructor trainee and not as a student, his mouth dropped. 'Are you crazy? Even healthy people sometimes have difficulty getting through this vigorous training program.' I continued to insist so finally he gave in and admitted me to the program through another back door.

"Once in the program, I believed that I was already a healthy person and followed the routine as much as possible. Although the teachers didn't know my weak condition when they admitted me, they soon found out when I had three near-death experiences during the first month of training. Fearing that I would die in their class, these teachers very much regretted my admission to the program.

"However, I was silently and stubbornly fighting my diseases during every training session. Each time I fell down, I would get back up on my feet; when I fell again, I would get up again. With tears and sweat, I would hang on to the practice without giving up. Finally, my teachers got the message that I was striving to live by working myself to death. They cheered me on. So with a strong will to live, I survived triumphantly. Not only did I win my battle against cancer, I also gained certification as an instructor. That was three years ago. This time I've come back to train more."

"Would you recommend people with severe illness to go through the same program?"

"No. My teacher was probably right in saying that I was crazy. People should go through the front door to learn Chi Lel."

I guess that anyone who is crazy enough to enter the back door deserves healing.

65. Sending Chi to Taiwan

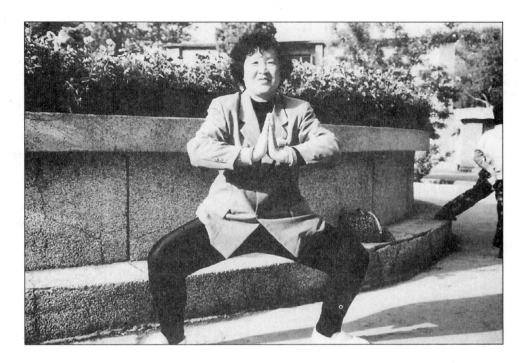

Chen Ai-Yun, 62, teacher

With her kind, caring attitude and bubbling personality, Teacher Chen is a natural teacher. She is in charge of a class of about sixty students who are mainly stroke victims. One day I went to her class and asked her students to raise their hands if they had gone through conventional hospitals before making their way to the Center. Almost everyone raised their hands. Then I asked those who felt that their condition had improved since doing Chi Lel to stand up. Everybody stood up except one man. When I later asked Teacher Chen about this particular student, she replied,"He just started two days ago."

"Teacher Chen, although you've only been teaching in the Center a year, you seem to have more experience than a lot of others. What is your secret?"

"Well, there's no secret. I was a healer in my hometown for many years before Lao-shi summoned me to the Center. I have facilitated the curing of several thousand people."

"How did you become a Chi-Lel healer?"

"I took up Chi Lel seven years ago. My life had been like a bowl of bad rice since 1966, the year the Cultural Revolution started. I was in and out of hospitals with a uterine tumor, a kidney infection, spleen problems, arthritis, dizziness, and insomnia. My family was held together by my husband as I was on and off work. Then in 1988 my dear husband died. His death was just too much for me to bear and I collapsed physically and mentally. It was during these dark days that a friend of mine encouraged me to take up Chi Lel."

"Did you believe Chi Lel would cure your ailments?"

"Not really. I joined our local Chi-Lel group for company and sympathy. At first, I had difficulty keeping up with the others because I couldn't stand up for more than a few minutes at a time. Fortunately, my teacher and everybody in our group understood my situation and gave me the love I needed to overcome my depression and other illnesses."

"How long did it take you to do that?"

"Half a year. Within that time, all the illnesses which had previously enslaved me finally left for good and I regained my youthfulness. Indeed, my life's script has been rewritten. The only regret I have is that my dear partner isn't here to share my joy. With newfound energy, I have begun to heal the sick and give them the same kind of love I had received when I was at the end of my rope."

"How about your family, do you help them when they are sick?"

"Definitely. I cured my daughter of her liver illness and gallstones and my grandson of his digestive problems. Also I sent chi to my big brother in Taiwan when I found out he had high blood pressure. Later he wrote me a letter saying that his blood pressure had returned to normal."

"How can you heal someone thousands of miles away?"

"Sending chi is not the same as sending electricity, which diminishes with distance. Chi exists everywhere simultaneously and can be used for healing. Every time I sent chi to my brother, I brought his image into our group as if he were in front of me. It worked."

66. A Faded Photograph

I stared at Teacher Zhang's youthful face in disbelief as she told me that she was sixty years old. Furthermore, she asserted that she had recovered from more than twenty illnesses. Seeing my amazement, Teacher Zhang showed me a faded photograph of herself taken almost thirty years ago. The picture showed her dark brown eyes resting in a hollow skull, staring into the camera. Her neatly combed hair and pretty dress couldn't cover the emptiness and suffering of a sick person.

"During the Cultural Revolution, my husband was branded as a 'poison weed' and our lives

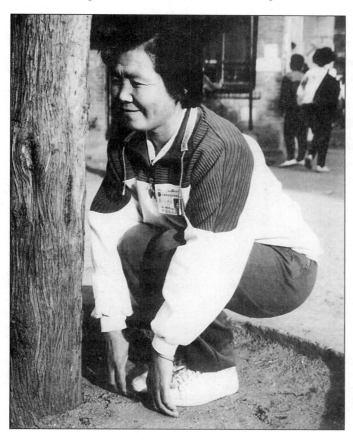

Zhang Sha-Zhi, 60, teacher

were turned upside down. Under such tremendous stress, I started to develop severe headaches, ringing in my ears, a running nose, and toothaches; I also had difficulty swallowing food. As time went on, my illnesses became more and more severe. I had kidney infections, an ulcer, spleen problems, arthritis, paralysis on the left side of my body, and an irregular heart rate.

"Were you very weak as a child?"

"No, I was a healthy child. Indeed, in school I was the envy of the other girls as I was an excellent sportswoman and a good singer. But in just a few years my illnesses turned me into an old woman who couldn't sing or walk. Wearing winter clothes year-round, I endured pain every day and moved as if I were walking on a layer of water. Indeed, my life was poisoned, and I was slowly choking to death."

"It must have been a very difficult time for you."

"Yes, it was and it became harder. Just as I thought I had seen the worst, my lungs contracted tuberculosis. Where before people hadn't cared about my illnesses because they were busy in their revolutionary activities, now I was despised and isolated because of my contagious disease. I stayed in the hospital for two and half years.

"Then the good news came that the Gang of Four had fallen into disgrace and my family was resurrected as being innocent. I was joyful as my mental pressure was released. However, my physical illnesses continued to plague me for another ten years."

"So when did you learn Chi Lel?"

"It was not until 1989 that I was introduced to Chi Lel and I have loved it ever since my first week of practicing it."

"What do you mean?"

"After the first week of practicing Chi Lel, my stomachache disappeared. With that encouragement, I began to take Chi Lel seriously by practicing the movements every day for long hours. It took me two years to conquer all my illnesses. Ultimately, four years ago, I became a teacher in the Center."

"Do you still practice Chi Lel seriously?"

"Absolutely, in battling my diseases, I mustn't let up. I still do the Wall Squatting two hundred times every day."

"Every day?"

"Yes, except one time. Last year I visited my son and he asked me, 'Mother, it's New Year's Day—won't you give yourself a day off?' The request seemed reasonable and I gave myself a day off. But I didn't feel too good that evening."

"Why not?"

"Well, you might think it was psychological but I realized that when I was having my day off my illnesses were working. If I don't take time to practice every day, eventually my illnesses will force me to take time off. So I would rather spend time on prevention now than spend time in convalesce later."

An ounce of prevention is certainly better than a pound of cure.

67. I Spent My Father's Gold Mine

In 1976 an earthquake hit the City of Tangshan in Northern China and killed or injured tens of thousands of people. One of the injured was Ms. Len, who was barely ten years old at the time.

"Even though my legs were injured during the earthquake, I was lucky to escape the calamity with my life," Ms. Len spoke softly as she relived her experience. "Many of my relatives were killed in their sleep when the horrible earthquake struck. I was terrified by the sight and smell of flesh."

"Were your legs badly hurt?"

"No, they didn't bother me at first because as a little girl, I expected myself to fully recover within a few days. But as days turned into weeks and weeks into months, the pain in my legs still didn't go away. Meanwhile, my joints became stiff and developed many bone spurs, creating more pain. I couldn't even roll over while laying down. When nature called, I couldn't bend my body to release myself. So I needed to wear split trousers, like a baby, to take care of my needs."

"Was your family supportive?"

"Yes, my father brought me to all kind of specialists including Western doctors, Chinese medicine doctors, and acupuncturists. Nothing seemed to help. Then last December I suddenly became paralyzed and was helplessly confined to bed for four months. While lying in bed, a relative gave me a videotape on Chi Lel. When I saw Lao-shi on the tape talking, I immediately felt chi. That night, as I watched the tape over and over again, I finally could get up! I mimicked some of the movements on the videotape and instantly felt life energy flowing in my spine. I was saved!

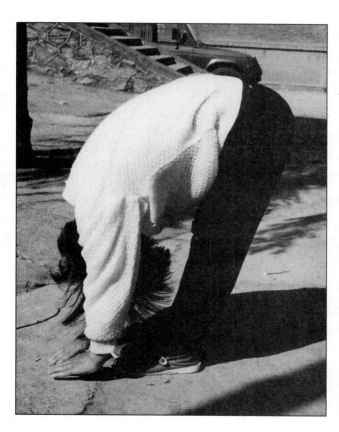

Len Shu-Hua, 29, student

"My father immediately sent me to the Center. Now I can bend my body and walk with my legs. Yes, I can walk! I am as free and happy as a bird! And all this happiness only cost me the price of a videotape. Yet, during the previous twenty years, I had spent more than 150,000 yuan on specialists. What a difference!"

"One hundred and fifty thousand yuan? That's a lot of money. Who had paid for it?"

"My father."

"What does your father do?"

"He mines gold."

"Really? Your family must be wealthy. I have heard that the Center needs funds for a Chi-Lel City. Do you think your father would be interested in donating some gold to support this cause?"

"Yes he would, if he finds another gold mine. I've already exhausted his first one." Ms. Len took her head, with much lamentation.

"Well, Ms. Len, I wish your father the best of luck in discovering another gold mine!"

68. Politically Correct

Ms. Geng was a government official before her illnesses forced her into early retirement. As an official, she was taught to be suspicious of anything unconventional and to report back to proper authorities on anything out of step with current beliefs. However, illnesses don't obey party lines and since conventional methods were ineffective, Ms. Geng was desperate for anything that could heal her.

"Even as a child, my legs had minor pains. These became more and more severe as I grew older. In my early forties, the forth and fifth vertebrae of my neck developed bone spurs and I couldn't even bend down to sweep the floor. Everyday I took six tablets of pain medicine to lessen my headaches and body pains. My blood pressure was low and I was prone to fainting on the street."

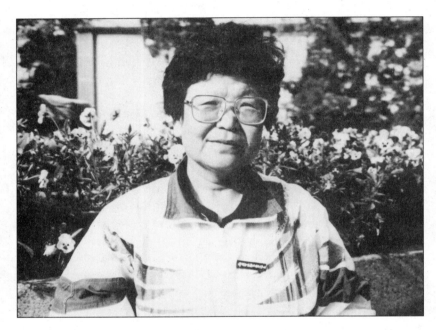

Geng Xin-Rong, 58, teacher

"What do you mean?"

"Sometimes I just fainted without any forewarning. One time I woke up on a street and wondered why so many people were surrounding me. Then it dawned on me that these curious people were looking at a stranger who had fainted while peddling her bicycle! As a strong government official, I bore my pain silently, but even with a strong will, I couldn't fight the sun."

"The sun?"

"Yes. In 1987, I suddenly became sensitive to sunlight. My skin would become itchy, swollen, and sore after exposure to the sun. So I would cover my body like an Arabian woman. Still it didn't work and I was forced into retirement. With the doctors unable to help me, I started to look around for a miracle."

"I thought, as a government official, you were not supposed to believe in miracles."

"True, that's why I used the word miracle, instead of 'reality.' I didn't believe qigong would work. One qigong 'master' promised that he would open my body channels if I gave him money. Well, if that were true, why didn't he open his sons' channels so that they could also become masters themselves? So I abandoned the idea of learning qigong.

"Then during my confinement I stumbled upon Lao-shi's book. It explained in simple terms that Chi Lel was not religion or quackery, but a new scientific frontier. The researchers of this frontier need to practice Chi Lel in order to understand it. In a sense every practitioner is a scientist exploring and discovering her own mystery. Being a scientist is a politically correct thing to do. So I began to practice Chi Lel with all my heart. After two months, I ventured out to practice under the sun. My whole body swelled but my skin wasn't itchy. After that my skin was no longer allergic to the sun. Furthermore, without paying attention to my spine, I discovered that I could bend my body close to my legs! Later, I began a second career as a teacher at the Center in May 1992."

"So is it politically correct to do Chi Lel, comrade?"

"It is, my brother."

69. A Soldier's Lonely Wife

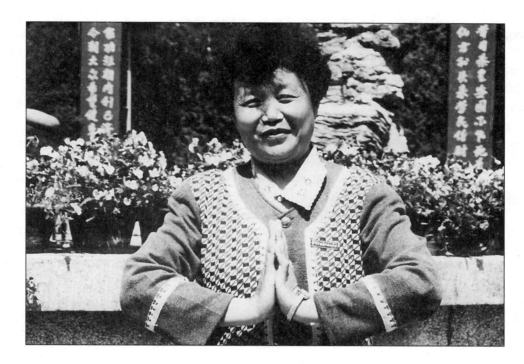

Yuan Xin-Mei, 48, teacher

Teacher Yuan was an accountant when she met her handsome army officer. They fell in love, married and had a daughter. Yet her husband had to live in the military compound while she lived with her mother-in-law at home. Teacher Yuan had to travel a great distance to visit her husband and life was lonesome and stressful with three generations living together under one roof.

Under such difficult conditions, Teacher Yuan developed insomnia, backaches, neuralgia, and severe headaches. "When the headaches attacked, I couldn't even open my eyes for days at a time. My body was so weak that a strong wind could have swept me away. I fainted easily and was afraid of walking alone."

"Did your mother-in-law give you any support?"

"No, in fact, she was the main source of my stress. She dominated every aspect of my life, leaving me no emotional outlet except crying. Indeed, I cried almost every night and became so anxious that people thought I was crazy. To me, life was a bowl of nervous worms."

"Was your husband aware of your situation?"

"Yes, because I cried each time I saw him. He understood my plight, but couldn't do anything about it. It would have been impossible for him to change jobs without our facing starvation and it would have been difficult to find new housing for my mother-in-law. So I suffered and each time my husband saw me my illnesses were worse than before."

"Did you seek help from professionals?"

"Yes, the doctors gave me a bunch of painkillers and sleeping pills. Although these medications helped me to some extent, they didn't actually heal me. Then my husband, during a visit with him in 1988, told me that he had taken up Chi Lel and encouraged me to do the same. 'But, my dear, how can you ask me to do something every day when I am not even motivated to get up in morning to face the world?' My husband replied, 'If you love me, you will try it.' 'Why are you taking it so seriously, my dear? Is it a love portion which will keep us loving each other forever?' 'It is more than love portion, it has cured my own intestinal afflictions and stomach-aches.'"

"So you took up Chi Lel immediately?"

"Not immediately, but the idea of taking up a daily exercise took root in my head. I started to pay attention to the people who were practicing Chi Lel in the park and finally joined them. The love I felt when I was with other practitioners was very therapeutic. After a few days I noticed the pains in my legs disappearing and, in two months, my headaches disappeared without a trace. Once more I felt the joy of life. My mind was so opened that I no longer regarded my mother-in-law as a liability. Of course, she also took up Chi Lel and we now practice the art together every day. We have become a harmonious and happy family again."

"Is your daughter also a Chi-Lel practitioner?"

"Yes, she has been practicing Chi Lel for two years. Moreover, being a medical doctor, she encourages her patients to take up the self-healing art so that they can recover faster."

"Why doesn't your daughter ask her patients to abandon the hospital in favor of self-healing?"

"Why should she? The two healing methods are complimentary, not contradictory to each other. Whatever works better for a patient should be recommended."

70. Helping Their Sons Take Examinations

"Our whole family practices Chi Lel every day and we make use of chi in an innovative way—we emit chi to our sons while they are taking their examinations."

"How do you do that, Teacher Sun?"

"While practicing Chi Lel at home, my husband and I bring life energy down from the universe to form a healing energy field around our sons who are in their classrooms preparing to take their examinations. We repeatedly say, 'Be calm, relax, have plenty of chi, answer questions correctly, and so on.'"

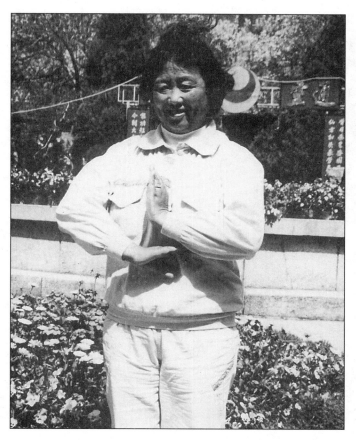

Sun Shu-Chong, 52, teacher

"Are you praying?"

"You might say that. However, we are not just saying good words, but also using our minds to deliver life energy to our sons. Because we have been doing Chi Lel for years, we can readily bring down chi from the sky for our use. As a result, all of our sons' report cards have showed good grades—good enough for them to get in the best universities. One of our sons has completed a medical degree and now studies in America, at Emery University in Atlanta—chi works!"

"Why do you have so much confidence in chi?"

"Because I have been transformed from a sickly to a healthy individual by the wonderful effects of chi. During the seventies, I had low blood pressure, anemia, and a low white blood cell count. In addition, I had stomachaches, female problems, kidney infections, and difficulty in walking. For me, life was a medicine bag which needed to be carried everywhere I went.

"Did you learn Chi Lel because the hospital couldn't help you?"

"Not really. I believed that the doctors had helped me a great deal in light of what they knew. Instead of looking around for other ways to better my life, I just accepted the fact that I was born to be sick. Then in 1987 my husband began doing Chi Lel because he was curious after watching so many people doing it."

"So you followed in your husband's footsteps?"

"It was not until many of his minor illnesses including a toothache disappeared after practicing Chi Lel that I decided to try it. Since my first lesson, I have never looked back. The more I practice, the more I feel the benefits of this amazing self-healing art. I love it, for besides curing all my illnesses, it has also helped me to develop special talents."

"What special talents?"

"Now I am working on a 'see-through' ability. Indeed, I can see through a person if I concentrate enough."

"Can you see through me?"

"Maybe next time—it takes a lot of chi. But let me show you how to see your own chi. Put your hands against a dark background and, squinting your eyes, look at the area in front of your fingers. Do you see some grayish white light coming out from your fingers?"

I squinted at my fingertips and replied,"Yes, I do."

"That's chi. Everybody has it."

That's it. Chi is so simple and yet so profound.

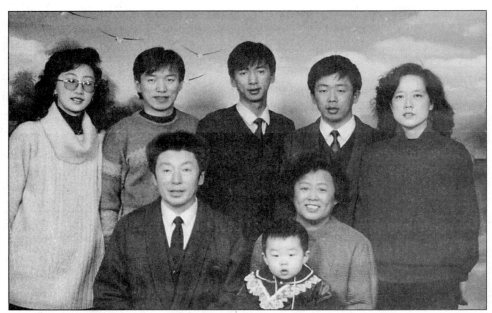

Teacher Sun and her family

71. The Man Who Likes To Drink Chi

At the age of sixty-five, Teacher Liu was as just energetic and enthusiastic as any young man at the Center, studying and teaching twelve hours a day.

"Look," he pointed to his hair, "since practicing Chi Lel, I have grown black hair and some of my wrinkles have disappeared."

"Do you practice Chi Lel to retain a youthful appearance?"

"Certainly not in the beginning. I was a sick man then. I mean I was a very sick man for a long, long time. From head to toe, I had twenty-four illnesses. I was dizzy and prone to black-outs because the blood vessels in my brain had hardened. I couldn't do much work because of high blood pressure and heart problems. I was thin and weak because of a ulcer. And furthermore, my ankles and knees were swollen with arthritis, which made walking difficult."

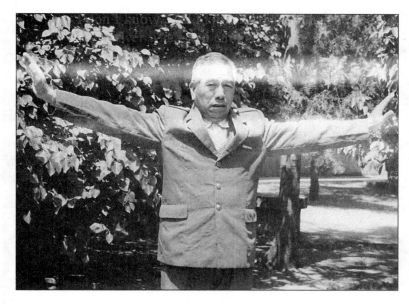

Liu Jiang-Fu, 65, teacher

"Did you take any medicines?"

"Yes, if I hadn't taken drugs, I wouldn't have been able to bear the pain. But if I took drugs to deal with one illness, they created another. Indeed, I spent all my years battling infirmities instead of enjoying life as a person should. How envious I was of those people who could walk freely, without pain. I longed for the day that I could be freed from my prison of disease.

"Seeing so many people practicing Chi Lel in the parks, I asked myself, if this exercise is not beneficial why are so many people doing it? Could all these people be crazy? The answer was obvious that I should try.

"Once I tried it, I felt as happy as a fish finding water. I practiced the art day and night until I forgot my own illnesses. Gradually all my ailments left me. I am now free of medication and can walk without pain or fear."

"Teacher Liu, it is difficult for many people to get rid of only one disease, let alone twenty-four. What's your secret?"

"I have no secret except to practice the art diligently. I practice the art even when I am not practicing the movements."

"What do you mean?"

"I have incorporated Chi Lel into my daily life. For example, when I drink a glass of water, I think the water is chi, good for my body. When I interact with people, I think we have formed a chi field, good for everyone."

"What if the people you are dealing with are negative, can you still form a good chi field?"

"Why not? You are the master of chi not a slave of it. You can form a healing chi field to benefit even the negatives."

"Is chi love?"

"I don't know. All I know is that chi has healed me and it is good."

His answer was good enough for me. So let's drink a glass of chi—the love of life!

72. Only a Three Day's Supply of Medicine

Ms. Wei was diagnosed with pancreatic cancer in August of 1994. She went to the hospital and got well for awhile. But when the disease reappeared she was hardly able to breathe and couldn't eat at all.

"How did you survive if you couldn't eat?"

"They kept me alive by intravenous feeding and I spent twenty-two days in the hospital. It was obvious I couldn't keep on living like that and doctors suggested surgery. I didn't want to go through surgery because the chance of recovery was small. My daughter is a nurse and she didn't advise me to go through the surgery either. On the other hand, my husband wanted me to go the Center."

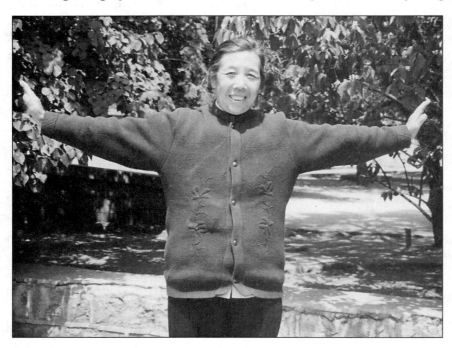

Wei Jin-Feng, 65, student

"Why did your husband want you to do that?"

"His chronic bronchitis had been healed by practicing Chi Lel for two years."

"You must have also been a practitioner?"

"No, I regret to say that I wasn't. I just didn't have the need to do the exercises then. But since I was at the end of my rope, I grasped Chi Lel as a last hope.

"Once at the Center, I practiced Chi Lel with all my heart. If I felt weak I still did the exercises in bed by imagining the movements. Now I can eat and sleep. Indeed, I have survived against all odds."

"By the way, how were you able to come to the Center if you couldn't eat?"

"My daughter is a nurse and we came here with only a three day's supply of medicine."

"Three days?"

"Three days, that's it"

"What if you hadn't responded to Chi Lel?"

"I don't know. I never had to face that."

Maybe Ms. Wei thought that in case of an emergency the Center would have been able to find some medicine for her. Or maybe she chose to burn all the bridges behind her in order to reinforce in her mind that the Center was her last hope and, by doing so, to summon her body and mind to work together in a final fight for her life. Whatever the case may be, I am still feel a sense of awe each time I think of her incredible story.

73. Being Without Money Was a Blessing in Disguise

Teacher Zhang is a beautiful young woman with a pleasant personality. She is one of the teachers on staff whose duty it is to teach students the Chi-Lel movements. While most of the young teachers have been healthy individuals all their lives, Teacher Zhang is an exception—she actually had been a 'student.'

"Four years ago, I had severe kidney problems and almost lost my life. I was hospitalized four times in one year, for up to two months at a time. Living in the countryside, my family didn't have the 'units' to pay my medical bills. So, in order for me to stay in the hospital, my parents needed to borrow money from relatives."

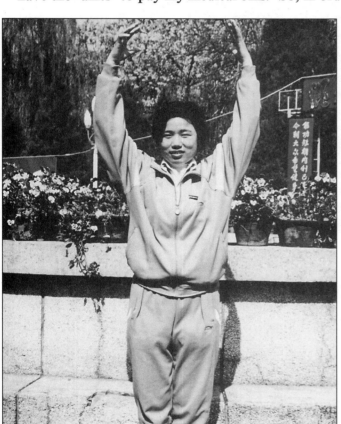

Zhang Ai-Xia, 23, teacher

"Can a hospital refuse treatment to a patient if he doesn't have money?"

"Sure. No money, no talk."

"How much money did your family borrow?"

"Ten thousand yuan. It was more difficult to borrow each time I went to the hospital because most of our relatives are poor, yet my illness was like a black hole, sucking in money as soon as it was received. Furthermore, my kidneys were like volcanos, ready to blow up anytime."

"So you dreaded the day the hospital would turn you away to die at home because you didn't have enough money to stay?"

"No."

"Why not?"

"Because each time I came home from the hospital, I thought I was cured and would never go back again. Still, my parents were worried to death."

"Then what happened?"

"One day my brother asked me to learn Chi Lel because a friend of his had been cured of cancer. At first I wasn't impressed because I believed that the city doctors knew best."

"What changed your mind?"

"Needles."

"What do you mean?"

"I was afraid of needles, which I'd had enough of while staying in the hospital, and I would have done anything to avoid them. So when my brother told me that Chi Lel was a natural healing method, with no needles or drugs, I jumped at the chance. I studied the method diligently and within a month, my kidneys were better. They continued to improve until they became normal again. My kidneys have not given me any trouble in two years."

"Teacher Zhang, if you had been a rich girl who could have afforded the hospital, do you think you would have chosen Chi Lel?"

"I don't know. For me, being without money was a blessing in disguise since I had no alternative but to do what I did. If I'd had money, I might have chosen to bear the pain of needles in a hospital, relying on others to cure me. I probably would have been proud of the fact that I could afford a hospital bed while others couldn't. But what kind of life would that have been to be bound to a hospital bed for life? Not much of a life. Don't you agree?"

"With all my heart."

74. His Pants Dropped In Front of Thousands of People

I first encountered Teacher Li when he was demonstrating in front of a class the power of chi by restoring a cracked raw egg back to its original form. The whole group including myself was amazed to see the cracked egg become to a perfect egg again. "Teacher Li, can you explain what's going on?" I asked.

"The theory of Chi Lel tells us that when chi gathers matter appears. When I heard that Chi-Lel teachers can gather chi to heal a broken limb in an instant, I began to experiment on eggs. Since eggshell and bones are both made of calcium, I believed that if I could heal a cracked egg I could do the same on a broken limb of a person. And it is a powerful visual demonstration of the nature of chi."

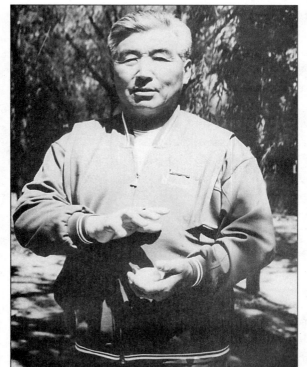

Li Ru-Chai, 62, teacher

"Why do you have so much faith in chi?"

"Chi saved me. I had suffered from many illnesses including asthma for forty years, high blood pressure and heart problems. I was on the verge of dying three years ago when my entire body swelled up and my head become as wide as my shoulders. Walking on crutches, I was a monstrous creature who couldn't lower his head to look down and couldn't sleep lying down. Doctors did all they could and I was left to die at home.

"My son had heard of the Center from a Chi-Lel practitioner and he brought me here. I was very fortunate that my son didn't give up on me and instead accompanied me to this healing place.

"Once at the Center, I instantly felt better because I was no longer treated as a patient but rather as an individual learning a self-healing art. All limiting thoughts such as 'my disease can't heal,' vanished. I began to practice Chi Lel diligently. One time I didn't sleep for seven days but continued to practice. I could hold my hands up at shoulder level for four and half hours."

"Why did you work so hard? Weren't you afraid that you would exhaust yourself and die?"

"I worked hard because I was afraid I would be defeated by disease. Yet death didn't terrify me anymore because my whole being, both body and mind, was busy fighting death and had no time left to be horrified by it.

"With persistence and single mindedness, I defeated my diseases and now I am acting as a teacher and cheerleader for those still struggling against theirs."

"I've heard that something funny happened to you when you shook hands with Lao-shi. Can you confirm this?"

"Yes, prior to meeting Lao-shi I was greatly overweight. However, when Lao-shi patted me on the back I lost twenty pounds in an instant! This caused my pants to fall down in front of thousands of people."

"Weren't you embarrassed?"

"Embarrassed for losing weight? No way!"

Indeed, chi works in funny, mysterious ways.

75. Her Boss Refused to Save Her Life—She's Glad

Speaking in a low, timid voice as though afraid of strangers, Ms. Liu told me that she had had bronchitis and stomach problems for thirty years. However, her voice rose as she spoke about her heart condition.

"Last year, I was hospitalized for two months for heart problems and doctors recommended immediate heart surgery. 'It would be the best way to put your heart at ease,' I was told.

"So I went to our unit to see my old boss for his approval. 'How much money will you need?' he asked.

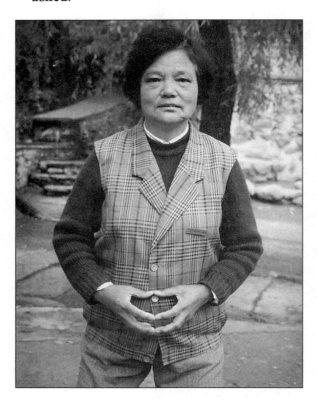

Liu Chong-Ru, 62, student

'Twenty thousand yuan.'

'We can't afford it.'

'Please sir, my heart needs it.'

'Sorry, I can't help you.'

'Don't you care?'

'I do, but if I give you the money, our unit will go bankrupt. Sorry.'

"I had worked for our unit all my life and now, when it had come down to money and death, I was left alone. Feeling betrayed, I went home and cried.

"With nowhere to turn, someone encouraged me to fight for my life by adopting a self-healing art. Luckily, I found Chi Lel and entered the Center last month. When I arrived here, I was so sick that I couldn't move or eat. But with hard work, love, and chi, I was nurtured back to health. Now I feel great and my heart is normal."

"Excuse me, Ms. Liu, how do you know your heart has been healed?"

"My body knows. My heart is beating normally and has no pain. Besides, an EKG has also indicated a well functioning heart."

"Congratulations, Ms. Liu. By the way, how much money have you spent here?"

"A few hundred yuan."

"You boss must be very happy to have paid a small amount of money to achieve a great result."

"He didn't pay a penny! I paid my own expenses."

"What do you mean?"

"It is our unit's policy to pay medical bills from only a few designated hospitals. The Center is considered outside this scope."

"So your boss left you to die because of lack of funds for your surgery, but didn't reimburse you even one penny when you found a way to help yourself?"

"Yes, on the one hand I should be angry, but, on the other, I am glad that he refused to save me. Otherwise, I probably would never have had the courage to take my health into my own hands."

"A blessing in disguise?"

"A blessing in disguise."

76. Kidney Stones in a Small Bottle

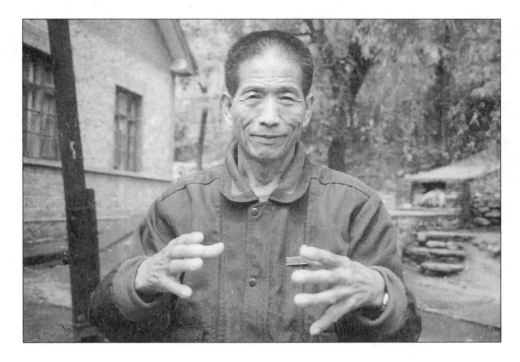

Yu Nai-Wen, 58, student

In 1985, Mr. Yu had two surgeries to remove kidney stones. Then six years later, he felt pain again and doctors discovered that his kidney had become misshapen because of five stones inside it.

"I couldn't believe it when the doctors told me that they couldn't operate on me because it would be too risky. What was I supposed to do? I asked them. They said that all they could do was to give me some medicine to take home."

"Did you go to another hospital for a second opinion?"

"Sure. I went to different Western doctors, herbalists, acupuncturists, and many other healers. They all shook their heads after charging me a fee. I spent a lot of money trying to get rid of my pain, which increased every day as the stones became bigger.

"Then four years later, I learned that my daughter's mother-in-law had recovered from a brain hemorrhage by doing Chi Lel. This was the first time that I actually believed that by doing some exercise I could heal myself."

"What do you mean by 'actually believed'?"

"You see, when I saw people exercising in the parks every day, I thought that they were just doing something for prevention or to just heal themselves of minor illnesses such as headaches or back pain, never kidney stones. But when someone I knew recovered from a more serious disease than mine by practicing Chi Lel, I became an absolute believer in the power of chi.

"So I came to the Center last month, and from the very beginning, I have practiced up to sixteen hours a day. When not practicing with our group, I would sit in a quiet place and do the La-Chi movements by opening and closing my hands."

93

"What did you think about while moving your hands?"

"I imagined my kidney ducts opening to infinity and the kidney stones going out."

"Did it work?"

"Yes. One night at nine o'clock, I went to the restroom to do the La Chi again. I said to myself repeatedly, kidney ducts expand, expand, expand and stones go down, down, down. Suddenly I felt sharp pain and knew something good was happening. Even though it was very painful I persisted, and finally at two o'clock in the morning, the kidney stones came out with my urine. What a big relief!"

"Is this true?"

"Yes," replied Mr. Yu. He took a small vial out his pocket and with a big smile said triumphantly, "Here. Five of them came out at one time!"

I congratulated Mr. Yu for doing something which no doctor could do for him. Then I remembered having seen two rows of small bottles filled with stones exhibited in the hallway with a label saying, "Friendship First, Competition Second!"

No wonder Mr. Yu had emphasized that his stones came out all at one time. There was a competition going on in which the goal was to reach a pain-free zone, but everyone who crosses the finish line will be a winner.

77. Deja Vu

Ms. Sun had had low blood pressure and a rapid heart rate of 124 beats per minute since she was in her early twenties.

"As I grew older, my heart gave me a lot of problems. Whenever I stopped taking medicine, my heart rate would increase rapidly. I always hid my medicine from my friends because they didn't understand how a young woman like me could be so dependent on drugs. How I longed to be as healthy as they were!"

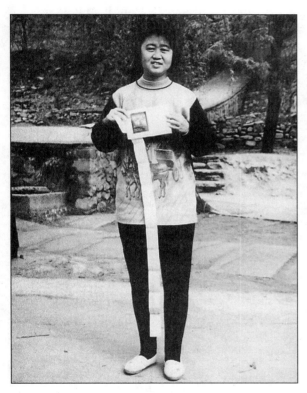

Sun Gui-On, 44, student

"Did you consider taking up a self-healing art?"

"No, I was reluctant to do any exercising for fear that it would send my heart rate out of control. I didn't want to disturb this beehive if I could help it, so to speak. Besides, I reasoned that if medication could suppress the symptoms, why should I try more? But then four years ago I was diagnosed with a uterine tumor.

"Doctors told me that surgery was the standard treatment for this type of tumor. Yet they hesitated to recommend surgery for me because of my weak heart."

"So what did you do?"

"Not much, just waited. Yet the doctors told me that my tumor was steadily growing. I felt like I was carrying a time bomb within me which was going explode at any moment. In this vulnerable state, I would have tried anything. So when a friend mentioned Chi Lel I was eager to try it."

"Did you really believe in Chi Lel?"

"No, not really, all of my life I had simply relied on doctors whenever I was sick. It never occurred to me that I could help myself in health matters. Otherwise I would have tried Chi Lel much earlier when I saw so many people practicing it in the parks.

"But this all changed when doctors were no longer able to help me and I was left on my own to fight for my life. Continued belief in my doctors would not save my life. In order to live I had to do something different, however fantastic. That's why I chose to come to the Center.

"When I arrived at the Center, I had a strange feeling that I'd been here before. My whole body seemed immersed in a great energy field and I felt an instant release. After two months of practice, my tumor was gone, as confirmed by two ultrasound examinations. My heart rate and blood pressure have also returned to normal."

"Do you still take any medicine?"

"No more. Twenty years is enough for me."

"What have you in your hands, Ms. Sun?"

"My EKG and an ultrasound diagram of my uterus. I am saving them as souvenirs."

"Are you happy now?"

"How could I not be?"

Indeed, there are a lot of happy people in the Center.

78. Saved By a "Future" Doctor

While his father did most of the talking, young Mr. Duan sat patiently next to me.

"My boy has had growth problems since he was small. The doctors believed it was his digestive system that was stunting his normal growth. He was hospitalized four times in 1991 for abdominal pain, but instead of getting better, his illness became more severe.

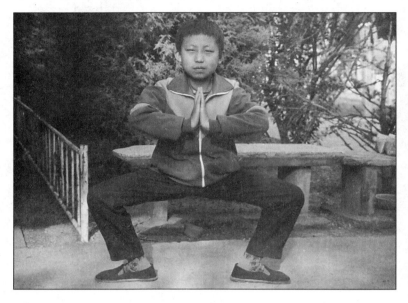

Duan Lun-Hui, 13, instructor trainee

"One day my son couldn't urinate and had to be hospitalized. The doctors surgically took out a stone as big as a grain of a corn from his bladder. Then we were told that it was my son's kidneys not his digestive system that were causing his growth problems!"

"Was this a relief to you?"

"Are you kidding? It was even more serious. The doctors tried laser surgery on his kidney stones, but that didn't work. Later they diagnosed him as having Fanconi's Syndrome and predicted that within five years his kidneys would be gone. And so would his life."

"Nothing could be done?"

"Nothing but wait for a medical breakthrough in my son's kidney disease. The doctors said he was too young to have a kidney transplant even if we'd had the money for the operation, which we didn't. So we resorted to herbal medicine."

"Did these medicines help?"

"No. Not only did they not help, they also messed up his stomach to the point where he vomited everything he took in, including food and water. Just when I thought he had reached the end of his rope, someone told us that there was a Western doctor helping people to help themselves."

"In a hospital?"

"Yes, the doctor treated my son, in a regular hospital, by emitting chi to him and teaching him Chi Lel. After five months of practicing Chi Lel, my son's kidney functions had returned to normal and he had grown both in height and weight."

"Can you tell me more about the doctor who prescribed Chi Lel to your son?"

"I was told that this doctor had healed his own eye disease by practicing Chi Lel, and so decided to treat patients in his spare time with Chi-Lel therapy. His reputation grew and many people came to see him. So the hospital assigned twenty beds for his special therapy."

"Only twenty beds?"

"Yes, but twenty was more than enough because the therapy emphasizes doing instead of resting, on 'self-service' rather than 'full service.' Some doctors in the hospital are taking note of this new model of treatment and have become practitioners themselves."

"So your doctor is some kind of 'future' doctor?"

"Yes, a future doctor now."

79. She Has Inspired 20,000 People

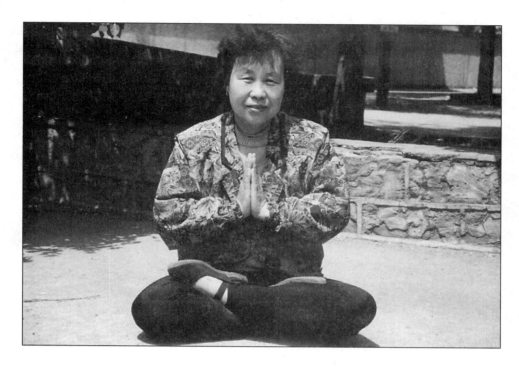

Bai Ching-Ming, 55, instructor trainee

When Ms. Bai told me that she had recovered from rheumatoid arthritis, I asked, "May I touch your hands?" With an understanding smile, she stretched her hands forward. I was amazed to find her hands very soft, like those of a youngster.

"But you can't touch my heart," Ms. Bai said jokingly.

"What do you mean?"

"I have also recovered from rheumatoid heart disease. In fact, I was so notorious for my illnesses that I was the number one patient in our unit."

"Why were you number one?"

"I had been in and out of hospitals for almost twenty years. In addition to arthritis and heart problems, my left kidney was atrophic and my right kidney misshapen. My blood pressure fluctuated between high and low and I had a degenerative joint disease in my spine.

"Everybody in our unit wanted me either to die or get well because I had spent so much of their money. Yet because I was young, my body tolerated the onslaught of different illnesses and hung on to life."

"Were you able to work?"

"No, I couldn't even walk and was always near an oxygen tank. We had to hire a maid to take care of me. Like most young people at the age of thirty, I had dreams and aspirations. But I lost all hope, and life became a prison of total dependency. I was dismally whirled about in a vicious cycle: sick-hospital-medicine-home-sick."

"No way out?"

"Not for twenty years until I made up my mind to help myself—to begin Chi Lel. Initially I

97

took up the exercise to keep my blood circulating so that my body would last longer. I dared not think that any self-healing art could heal my illnesses."

"How were you able to practice in your condition?"

"I started just moving my hands while sitting and gradually progressed to doing the movements in a standing position. After a month's practice, my spirits returned and I felt hope. Getting up at four in the morning every day, I was eager to do the exercises. Then one day I heard myself asking, 'Why am not I feeling pain when it snows?' Immediately, as if a huge life energy ball were pouring from the sky, my whole being was infused with joy.

"With hope, I continued to do the exercises day and night. At one point, I vomited a lot of blood, but didn't go the hospital. At another time, my legs turned almost black and itchy. But I was not concerned and continued to practice, practice, and practice. Gradually, from a mere eighty pounds, I gained until I was back to my normal weight of 120 pounds. After half a year's practice, I was finally freed from the bondage of illness and once more the light of life shone on me.

"Because my medical history was well documented, even some of the worst critics of self-healing arts have become believers. It is estimated that 20,000 people had taken up Chi Lel because of my case and our unit has saved a lot of money as a result."

Ms. Bai endured incurable illnesses for twenty years, but her sufferings have not been in vain.

80. A Predictable Headache

When Ms. Li turned twenty-one she discovered that she had a predictable headache—from 9:00 am to 11:00pm every day. This headache would plague her for the next twenty-seven years.

"Each day, at the onset of my headache, I would take six painkillers. My memory was so bad that at times I forgot whether it was day or night."

"Headache and loss of memory only?"

"No, other diseases followed. All my internal organs, except my pancreas and spleen, were sick at one time or another. My illnesses included high blood pressure, coronary disease, kidney disease, stomachaches, liver problems, intestinal infections, and tuberculosis. In addition I had problems with the blood vessels in my brain and my whole body had degenerative joint disease.

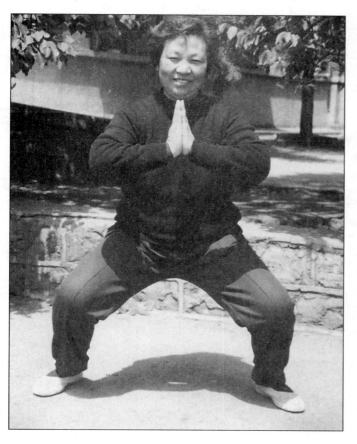

Li Hua-Ting, 57, instructor trainee

"Even though I sought help from the best hospitals, my life was without hope because the doctors were just as helpless as I was. At night, I could only sleep in one position and if I turned accidentally, I wouldn't be able to get up the next morning and would require hospitalization. So someone was always around to keep an eye on me. My life was just a bowl of pain."

"Why didn't you take up an exercise to help yourself? Didn't you see people practicing qigong in the parks every day?"

"Yes, everyone who has eyes can see thousands of people doing exercises in the parks. But since I was under doctors' care and they didn't advise me to look into any self-help methods, I never dared to do something like that. So like a frog being cooked slowly in hot water, I didn't have enough motivation to get out my plight.

"Then one day I heard an enthusiastic neighbor talking about his experiences with Chi Lel. I became fed up with my sufferings and ventured to do something different about my situation. With a new attitude that I could be helped, I began Chi Lel. Even after just one practice session, I could fall into a sound sleep without the aid of sleeping pills! With such a powerful signal that this self-healing art would cure my illnesses, I plunged into the practice.

"After a few months, all my illnesses were gone, including my long time companion—my headache. And I don't miss it!"

"What have you been doing since your recovery?"

"What else? Promoting Chi Lel. I want all the frogs being cooked in hot water to jump! jump! jump! out of the cooking pot into a free, cool, and beautiful pond."

Thanks Ms. Li, we have heard you loud and clear.

81. Thrice, My Skull Didn't Crack Like A Nut

Ten years ago Mr. Wang developed persistent headaches and loss of memory. After an occasion when he fainted and was brought to the hospital, doctors discovered that his brain was atrophic with three vascular blockages on the right side.

"My life changed dramatically. I couldn't remember things anymore and I reacted to things very slowly as though I were retarded. With no strength, I was afraid to venture out of our house.

"Even with extreme caution I fainted three different times but luckily, my skull didn't crack like a nut. From 1986 to 1990 I was hospitalized four times. Each time doctors put me on a CT, and each time they found my condition either hadn't improved or had worsened after medical treatment.

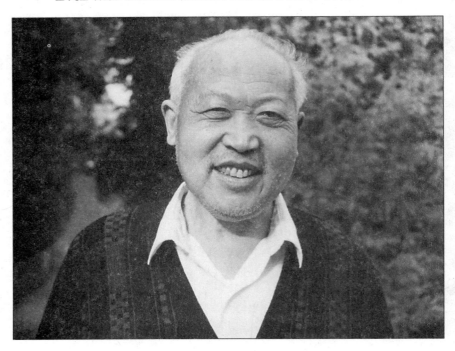

Wang Wing-Guang, 71, instructor trainee

"Meanwhile my wife was hospitalized for coronary disease, stomach problems, and white spots inside her mouth. The hospital couldn't do much for her either.

"Since we had nowhere to turn, my wife and I reached the decision that we should take up some ancient recipe—some self-healing art. After four months of Chi Lel, my wife had recovered. Her oxygen tank, still lying at home, has not been used since."

"How about yourself?"

"After eight months of hard and dedicated work, I also recovered. I can still see my doctor's puzzled face as he looked at the CT results—a normal brain. A miracle happened! Having almost lost my brain, I had now had reclaimed it. What a relief!"

"Are you still doing Chi Lel?"

"Absolutely, my wife and I practice it daily."

"What's your purpose for doing Chi Lel now?"

"For prevention and also for fun. We feel so good after practicing Chi Lel that it is beyond description. It is an art that improves with age. We look forward to our daily practice ritual because we know that each day we are getting better at it. We feel young and we love it."

"In other words, you and your wife are still learning and growing every day?"

"Every day."

At the age of seventy-one, Mr. Wang and his wife are still are not yet over the hill because they are still climbing up the hill.

82. Goodbye Wheelchair, Hello Freedom

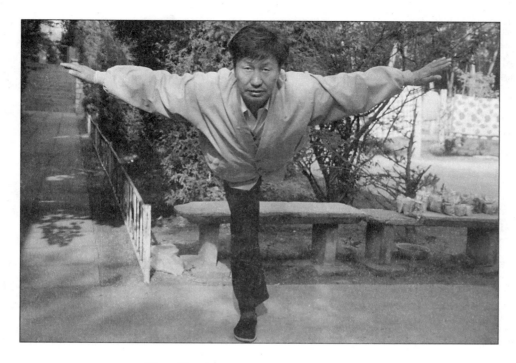

Han Sho-Tian, 59, instructor trainee

Mr. Han already had a fractured right hip and a degenerative spine before he suffered a stroke which paralyzed the right side of his body in September of 1983.

"The doctors told me to rest a lot, and, because of high blood pressure, to avoid being angry, worrying, or doing anything that might trigger another attack."

"Could you walk?"

"No, I could hardly move and was confined to a wheelchair. My right leg began to shrink and became obviously smaller than my left leg. And not only did I lose body movement, but also speech and memory skills. My family and friends were surprised to hear me murmuring nonsensical questions like, 'What degree? Does temperature have degrees?' Indeed, I became a total dependent who needed assistance even to eat and dress.

"When I returned to the hospital for a checkup, I saw many others like myself, in wheelchairs being pushed by family members. A chill ran up my spine as I overheard one of them saying that he had been in wheelchair for more than ten years after a stroke. What kind of future was I looking forward to? Depressed, I went home and cried silently to myself.

"Then one day a visiting friend told me about Chi Lel and taught me to move my good hand to collect chi. 'If you can't move much, make up for it by using your mind,' he told me. Immediately I learned to move my left hand to deliver chi to my body. From morning till night, I poured chi into myself, thinking that chi was arriving and that my illnesses were disappearing. It might seem crazy, but I was doing something for myself and I felt the power of life energy working on me. When pain appeared I told myself, it's good, and continued to practice even more.

"Sensations in the paralyzed part of my body began to return. After about a hundred days of practice, I could walk with a crutch; after half year, I could walk freely. Now I have been normal for the past ten years."

"So good-bye wheelchair and hello freedom?"

"Yes, liberation and no wheelchair!"

"Mr. Han, people have various reasons for being confined to wheelchairs, do you think Chi Lel can help all of them?"

"Certainly, chi works wonders. However, one must have persistence and confidence. Sometimes it is very frustrating when nothing happens for a long period of time. During these times, one must 'foolishly' hang on to Chi Lel. The final victory belongs to those who have faith."

"How were you able to have so much faith?"

"I had no choice but to believe it would work. The alternative was just unthinkable."

"So you wouldn't accept a fate of being confined to a wheelchair for life?"

"Who said it was my fate not to be able to walk again? I believe I can walk and now I am walking. That's my fate!"

When belief is combined with chi, miracles happen.

83. Misfortune Dropping From the Sky

At age of thirty-seven, Mr. Zhang was a normal, healthy man. Then one day while he was walking down the sidewalk, a board fell from above and hit him.

"Out of the blue, I was hit in the head by some debris while going to work. Since the impact didn't cause any bleeding or great discomfort, I dismissed the episode as 'just not my day' and went to work as usual.

"Yet without my knowing it, the blood vessels in my brain had been damaged, affecting my brain and causing the left side of my body to be paralyzed."

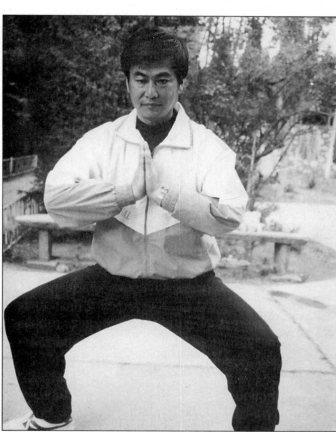

Zhang Xu-Zhou, 45, instructor trainee

"Just like that?"

"That was it, half of my body gone. The doctors couldn't do much to improve my situation and told me that the best I could hope for was to remain where I was the rest of my life."

"How long did the doctors treat you before giving up?"

"Eight months. After that I took herbal medicine for awhile, but that didn't help either. With nowhere to turn, I felt hopeless. I was terrified to think of my young family."

"So you were in a wheelchair, feeling depressed?"

"I wish. I couldn't even sit in a wheelchair! But just when I was beginning to give up hope, I read an article about Chi Lel. This article, which mentioned many people who had recovered from incurable illnesses by practicing this self-healing art, was incredibly attractive. If I hadn't reached a dead-end road, I probably would have dismissed the article as too good to be true. But with my situation as it was, I would have tried anything which promised even the slightest possibility of recovery.

"Before I went to the Chi-Lel class, I was a bit apprehensive about the whole thing. Would people laugh at me? Would people take me in only because I was in such a vulnerable condition? But when I met my teacher and classmates, all my doubts vanished as I felt the love and understanding from everybody.

"Instead of treating me as incurable, my teacher taught me to move my hands to collect chi and told me that as long as I practiced diligently I would recover soon. Empty talk? Well I didn't sense any hypocrisy in her voice. Indeed, my teacher's sincerity in speech and action instilled in me a new belief—a belief that I could muster my own healing energy for recovery. My new belief became so strong that it overcame the old conditioning of seeing myself as being a cripple-for-life."

"Did your teacher have such magical power to instill belief?"

"My teacher, like any good teacher, could only do so much for her students. I listened to her and diligently practiced Chi Lel, which helped me to regain feeling in my hands and shoulders. Feeling improvement, my belief and confidence skyrocketed and I practiced even more. With more practice, I finally could stand up and walk!"

"How long did it take you?"

"Three months from the time I practiced in bed to standing up and walking free. Of course, each individual is different. Some take a year or even longer. But one thing is sure: the more effort one puts into practice the sooner one recovers."

"How long has it been since you regained your freedom?"

"Five years."

"Still practicing Chi Lel everyday?"

"Yes, practicing Chi Lel is more important than sleeping or eating."

"What do you mean?"

"I could do without sleeping or eating for a day or two but not Chi Lel. By practicing Chi Lel, I gain life for my daily activities."

84. I Took Chi Instead Of Medicine

After Ms. Zhuo was diagnosed with lung cancer, she was hospitalized for seven months. While still in the hospital, her cancer began to spread and consequently doctors removed a quarter of one of her lungs. However, following the operation and two doses of chemotherapy, Ms. Zhuo's lung condition had not improved and she was unable to eat.

"Then one morning, I encountered an old friend in the park. She told me that her year-round cold had been cured after practicing Chi Lel for a short time. She encouraged me to do the same saying, 'You look so awful.'

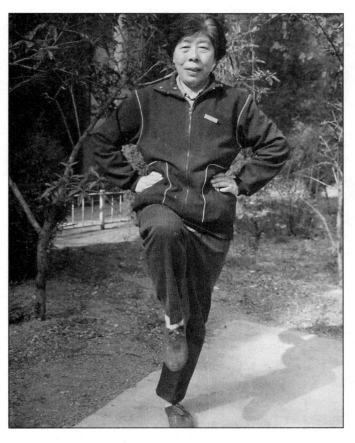

Zhuo Yong-Gui, 61, instructor trainee

"I knew this friend well—she had always been a sick person. But seeing is believing and I could see that she had been transformed into a spirited and healthy individual. So I decided to take up the self- healing art."

"You had a much more serious illness than your friend. Why were you so sure Chi Lel would help you?"

"I had no choice but to believe in something because chemotherapy was not helping me. So I took Chi Lel seriously and, after practicing for half a year, my cancer disappeared along with my high blood pressure and coronary disease. I was given a second chance in life."

"How do you know your lungs are cured?"

"A year ago I went back to my doctor for a CT and ultrasound examination. He was surprised to find a healthy lung, asking, 'Have you been taken my medicine?'

'No.'

'Why not?'

'I have been taking chi instead.'

'You didn't even take some medicine for strength?'

'No. It cost too much.'

"My doctor laughed and asked me to give him the information about Chi Lel."

"How much money did you spend on hospital care?"

"Forty thousand yuans, with no result."

"How much have you spent on Chi Lel?"

"Two hundred yuans, with a happy result."

"What a difference!"

"Do you mean the result or the amount of money?"

"Well, both I guess."

85. Tree of Sweat and Tears

In her early forties, Ms. Yu's health took a dive. She developed high blood pressure, coronary disease, gallstones, kidney problems, stomachaches, and rheumatoid arthritis.

"Other than my lungs, all my body functions were bad," Ms. Yu began. "Every specialist in the hospital knew me by name as I regularly took turns seeing them. After being in and out of the hospital for about ten years, I suddenly developed blockages in the blood vessels of my brain, which caused half of my body to become paralyzed. This was the last straw in my already hopeless situation, as doctors predicted that I would soon become totally paralyzed."

"So what did the doctors tell you to do?"

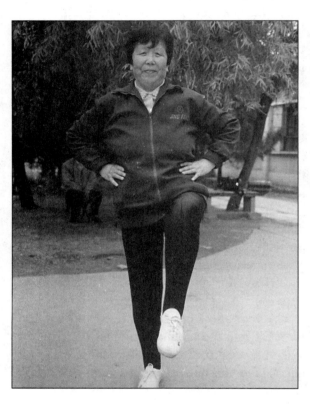

Yu Xun-Lan, 63, instructor trainee

"They told me to get plenty of rest, eat whatever I liked, and wait until science found a cure for my ailments. They assured me that if man could walk on the moon, there wasn't any reason that man couldn't come up with something to deal with my problems. 'But how long will it take?' I asked them.

"With little hope, I arranged for my burial and waited for heaven to take me. While I was vegetating at home, a friend told me about Chi Lel. Sensing my excitement during his descriptions of some incredible cases of healing, my friend warned, 'The prescription for Chi Lel is plenty of hard work, not plenty of rest. If you take up Chi Lel you will enter into a war against your diseases. Are you afraid?'

'Since I am already dead what can I be afraid of? When can I join your group?'

'I'll teach you some movements now.'

"This friend introduced me to Chi Lel then and there and I have loved it from the first movement. Since I couldn't walk, I needed to be carried to the group practice. Every morning I got up at four o'clock to finish my three to five hours of daily practice.

"At first I needed to do the movements near a tree so that I could hold onto it if I fell. With the tree as my companion, I battled my pain in sweat and tears. Each time I squatted down the pain was excruciating. Yet after each struggle I felt better and proud of myself. Finally I was doing something to fight back at my diseases and I felt satisfaction in being able to throw some punches head on—pain against pain."

"What do you mean by pain against pain?"

"I created pain as a result by defying my diseases' wishes for me to stay home, resting. Yet such pain was required to overcome my illnesses. After twenty days of practice, I had stopped taking my daily medicine and found I could walk slowly. And after three months my health had basically returned to normal. Now after ten years of daily practice, I am better physically and mentally than many people my junior."

Indeed, with Ms. Yu's smooth face and robust body, no one could dispute her claim.

86. A Japanese Girl Said Good-bye to Her Hearing Aid

Ms. Wang, a child of a mixed marriage between a Japanese mother and a Chinese father, was born and raised in Japan. When she was two years old, she lost her hearing because of a high fever. Living in Japan, she could afford the latest medical tool—a hearing aid. But her father did not want his daughter to wear hearing aids all her life, so he brought her back to China, to the Chi-Lel Center.

"How long have you been in the Center?"

"Four months," Ms. Wang replied in perfect Chinese.

Then I turned to her teacher and asked,"Since Ms. Wang is from abroad, and accustomed to a living standard which is much higher than that in the Center, does she get special treatment?"

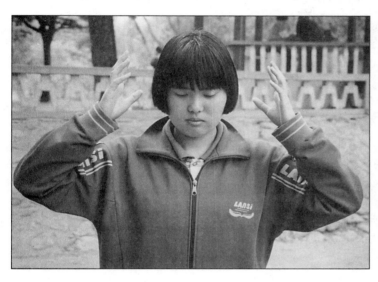

Wang Ching, 18, student, with the author

"No, we don't have special facilities for foreign guests. We are planning to build a Chi-Lel City in the future so that more people from abroad can come here."

"Ms. Wang, do you feel comfortable here?"

"Yes. Although in the beginning it took some effort to adjust to the living tempo here, with the support and care of my teacher and fellow students, I settled down and am now practicing Chi Lel diligently."

"How long had you been wearing your hearing aids?"

"As long as I could remember. Even after three months in the Center, I was still wearing my hearing aids every day."

"Why?"

"Because I was afraid people would think that I was a retarded person. People who didn't know me would think I couldn't understand their words.

"Then one morning my teacher asked me, 'Why don't you take off your "things" while practicing?' Being an obedient student, I took off my hearing aids. As soon as I had unplugged the 'things' I was startled to find myself hearing just as well as I had with the hearing aids. Was I dreaming? I shook my head and touched my ears again to see if I had another pair of hearing aids on. No, I wasn't wearing any and I could hear perfectly. Oh! I could hear!"

"Just like that?"

"Yes, just like that—no needles, no medicine," Ms. Wang replied, smiling sweetly.

Even though Ms. Wang didn't have the courage to take off her"things" for three months, the power of chi had worked on her nonetheless.

Most people have many priorities in their lives, as did Ms. Wang. Yet she was willing to give up all her activities for a few months to go through a vigorous training program in a self-healing art. Was the result worth the effort? Maybe some people are willing to bear their inconvenience of wearing a hearing aid instead of"wasting" their time trying to heal themselves. Yet for a young woman like Ms. Wang, regaining her hearing provided a great boost to her self-esteem. The joyful smile on her face told it all.

107

87. Sixth Floor? No Problem!

Mr. Wang was the chief engineer in his unit, a petrochemical concern. Over the years he developed a high blood pressure and coronary disease and was on medication for many years.

"The first attack came last February when my heart suddenly stopped beating for five to thirteen minutes; then I was hospitalized for more than a month. The second attack came six months later as I woke up shaking with my heart beating irregularly. Once again, I was hospitalized for another month."

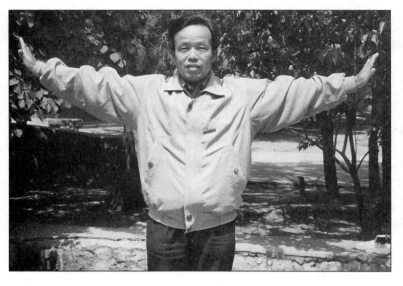

Wang Zhao-Jiang, 56, student

"Were you able to work after hospitalization?"

"No, after an occasion when I found myself immobilized on the street after walking for less than thirty minutes, I told myself, That's it. I am not going anywhere anymore. I was even afraid to go outside of my house because my heart, like an active volcano, could erupt anytime. So I became a prisoner in my own home."

"When did you begin Chi Lel?"

"About a month later, when a friend told me about it. At first I doubted if I could do it and asked my friend, 'If I can't even walk without panting, how can I expect to stand forty minutes at a time?'

"My friend explained, 'In practicing Chi Lel, you are not expending energy like other sports such as jogging or playing basketball, instead you are absorbing life energy. So one can stand for a long time without feeling exhausted. Try it for yourself.'

"I tried and found the more I practiced the more I could absorb life energy, which, like soft raindrops on young plants in the springtime, nourished my body and mind.

"After four months of practice, my heart functions had returned to normal, which was confirmed by doctors using an EKG. Now I can go anywhere I want. Once I called a friend to tell him that I was going to pay him a visit. Being a kind and concerned individual, my friend said, 'Let me visit you instead. My house is on the sixth floor and there is no elevator.'

"'Sixth floor? No problem!' I laughed hung up the phone. An hour later I showed up at his doorstep. My friend was so surprised to see me well and healthy that, after inquiring about Chi Lel, he took it up immediately. It's wonderful that my friends are also getting benefits from practicing Chi Lel."

"Excuse me Mr. Wang, your heart has just recently been healed. Aren't you afraid your old condition might come back?"

"It is always possible that I might have heart problems again. But if that occurs, I'll treat it as a new disease because my old illness has been cured. I'll fight the new one as I have done before. In fact, by practicing Chi Lel every day, I am nipping any new enemies in the bud even before they have a chance to grow into horrible shapes."

In his war against diseases, Mr. Wang had found an easy and efficient battle plan—fight them before they come into existence.

88. The Latest Victim of World War Two

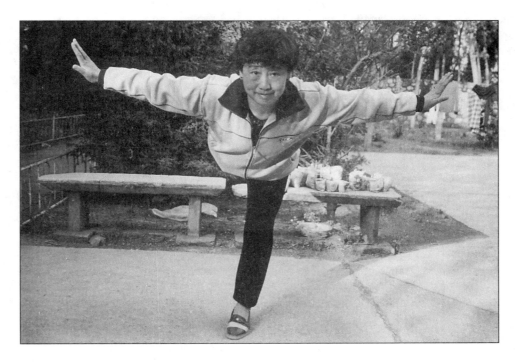

An Jun-Feng, 46, instructor trainee

When Ms. An told me that hot blood had come out of her body, I didn't understand what she meant.

"I was a victim of hemorrhagic plague."

"Do you mean black plague, the disease spread by rats?"

"Yes."

"How come?" I was surprised, thinking that this disease had disappeared long ago.

"The doctors told me that during the World War Two the Japanese had released some infected rats as an experiment on human beings. People in my area still catch this disease and I am one of them."

"Were you bitten by a rat?"

"No, I don't know how I contracted the disease, but I also had a legacy of kidney, stomach, joint, throat, heart and brain problems. Since 1988, I had been hospitalized regularly two or three times a year."

"Were you working at the time?"

"No, I wasn't able to work. Then in 1992, my heart became so weak that it couldn't pump enough blood to supply my body, including my brain. The blood vessels in my eyes were hardening, causing my vision to worsen each day. When I was sent to the best hospital in the big city, the doctors were surprised to find so many ailments in one body and said, 'One illness at a time. Be patient, we can't treat them all at once.'

"Somehow I became disillusioned about these big-city doctors because they should have been honest with me about the fact that I couldn't be helped. How could they treat one illness without affecting the other? Even if they were able to fix one part of my body, how did they know my whole body would be healed? In fact, I was more familiar with my own illnesses than many of the doctors. For them, the treatment of my diseases was no more than a job, nothing personal; but for me, defeating my diseases meant life or death."

"What did you do about your situation?"

"Nothing but despair. Luckily my brother told me about Chi Lel because he had heard of someone having been cured of a serious heart disease by practicing it. But, he warned, 'It takes hard work and you are as sick as a dog.'

"I knew I'd be all right, because, before my illnesses, I had been a hard worker all my life. Besides, I was only forty-three and sick and tired of being pushed from one hospital to another. It was time for me to say, 'Enough is enough, I am fighting back.'

"So I began Chi Lel with all my heart. Instead of feeling alone and helpless when confined in my sickbed, I was strengthened by a group spirit as my teacher and classmates helped me and cheered me on. Indeed, I was no longer a patient at the mercy of my illnesses but a gallant soldier fighting my deadly enemies one trench at a time. After three months of practice, I had recovered. When I returned to work, our unit chose me as a model worker."

"Model worker? I thought you hadn't worked for awhile."

"That's true. But I was a model worker for saving our unit money."

"How?"

"By not being sick."

Indeed, Ms. An had inspired many workers to take up Chi Lel, saving her unit much money.

89. Dear Husband, Please Don't Abandon Me Because I Am Sick

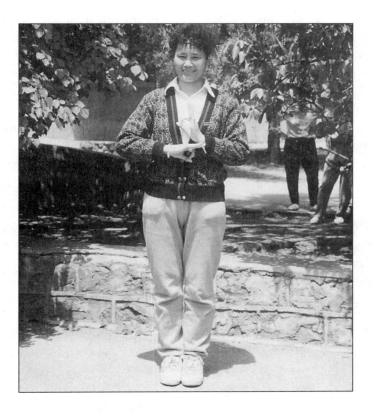

Lou You-Fang, 44, instructor trainee

For many years, Ms. Lou had irregular heartbeats, diarrhea, and a severe headache which incapacitated her every afternoon at four o'clock. Then in May of 1994, doctors diagnosed her as having stomach cancer and operated immediately to remove it.

"I was a weak person before and was even weaker after the surgery—I fainted easily and could hardly walk. When doctors followed up my surgery with chemotherapy, I couldn't stand the chemical that was injected into my body. But when my husband suggested I should abandon chemotherapy in flavor of Chi Lel, I was deeply hurt."

"What do you mean?"

"I thought my husband was trying to get rid of me. We had bitter arguments and I begged him not to abandon me when I was sick. But he insisted, saying, 'You know that chemotherapy is killing you. Chi Lel is your only chance.'

"But I argued, 'Husband, you just want me to die so that you can marry a healthy woman, don't you?'

'No, we have gone through many ups and downs in our lives. I haven't abandoned you before and I am not about to do it now.'

'If it is so, why do you want me to give up the best medicine available in the world in flavor of some medicineless, wishful-thinking, self-help kind of exercise?'

'Because Chi Lel is good for you and I care about you.'

'Please don't sugar your real intention in the name of caring about me. Let me ask you, when you are sick, do you go to the hospital or to the park?"

"My husband remained silent after I poured out my frustration on him. Meanwhile I knew that

111

Chi Lel was the only option left, whether I liked it or not.

"So I registered at the Center and began my self-healing journey. After three months, I was a free person again because not only was my cancer gone, but also my diarrhea and the enslaving four-o'clock headache. Meanwhile, I received a registered letter from my husband, telling me that he missed me and that he had sent money, six thousand yuan, so that I could get a maid to serve me. Tears came to my eyes as I finally realized that my husband did indeed love me very much."

"What would have happened if your husband hadn't suggested you take up Chi Lel?"

"I don't know. But one of my co-workers who had cancer similar to mine died."

"How did your husband come up with the idea that you should take up this healing art and, by doing so, avoid the same fate as your co-worker?"

"He always had sense. Maybe that's why I married him in the first place," Ms. Lou replied with a smile.

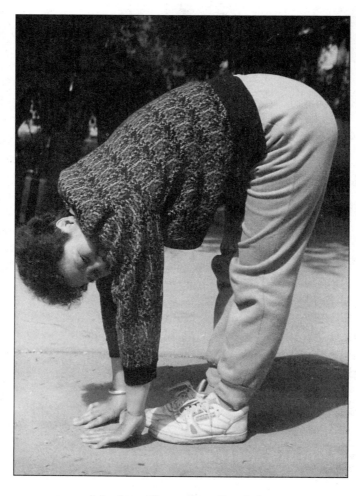

Ms. Lou Shows her flexibility

90. Does My Boyfriend Truly Love Me?

When Ms. Zhen, an attractive lady of twenty-five, began to experience persistent abdominal pain, she went to see a doctor. The doctor told her that she had a 5x5 cm tumor in her right ovary.

"It hit me like thunder on a sunny day because I had always been a healthy person and never expected that I would become sick. The doctor went on to advise me to avoid vigorous exercise such as jumping which could stimulate the growth of the tumor.

"I asked him, 'Doctor, are you telling me to maintain a quiet lifestyle when I have been active been all my life?'

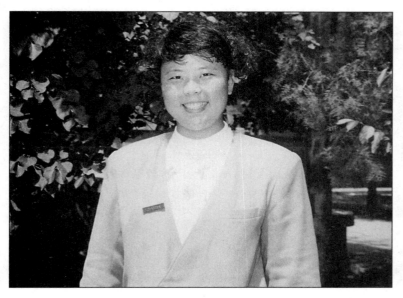

Wang Zhao-Jiang, 56, student

'Yes, and if you want to have a child later on, you must follow my advice. When your child is due, it can only be delivered through a C-section operation. After that your ovary will need to be removed and you won't be able to bear any more children. By the way, do you have a boyfriend?'

'Yes?'

'The sooner you marry and become pregnant the better your chances of having a child in your life.'

'But doctor, I am not even sure if my boyfriend truly loves me. How can I rush into things?'

'That's your choice,' the doctor replied and left me alone.

"Did you get a second opinion?"

"No, instead I went to my family for advice. My mother and big sister assured me that Chi Lel could help me."

"Did they practice Chi Lel?"

"Yes, everyone in my family except me had taken up Chi Lel after my mother healed herself of a heart condition. Indeed, my little sister was in a Chi-Lel instructors' training program at the time."

"Why didn't you practice Chi Lel before?"

"Like many other young people, I guess I didn't have the need or discipline to do those slow and gentle exercises. Instead I spent my time on bowling, jogging, dancing, and other active sports. Sometimes I thought my sisters were behind the times by doing something a thousand years old. Yet when I was in trouble my sisters became my heroines. They helped me and encouraged me to practice Chi Lel. Just after a month's practice, my tumor was gone!"

"During this trying period, did you find out whether your boyfriend truly loves you?"

"Yes, he does love me very much," Ms. Zhen replied with her face turning red. "He even emitted chi to me."

"So he will be your mate for life?"

"Maybe, but now I am not in a hurry to choose a mate."

A true love can wait.

91. If I Should Die On the Train, So Be It!

Ms. Xiang, a school teacher, underwent surgery for intestinal cancer in December 1992. After two years of chemotherapy, the cancer, instead of disappearing, had spread to her left kidney. The doctors recommended removing her kidney in order to contain the cancer.

"The doctors told me that by sacrificing one of my kidneys, I could save my life. I asked if there were risks involved, and they said yes. 'But this is the best option for you right now.'

"Meanwhile someone told me about Chi Lel and its curative effects. But I wasn't convinced because I believed the doctors knew best. So I decided to let go of my cancerous kidney and when it was gone, I thought so were my sufferings.

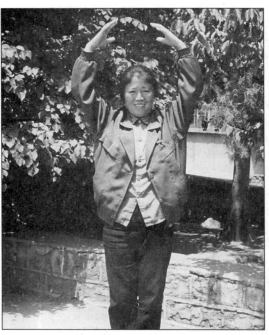

Xiang Qiao-Li, 40, student

"But three months later, bad news came again as the doctors found cancer in my bladder. They couldn't operate on me anymore because I was too weak. Chemotherapy remained as the only weapon the doctors had against my cancer. But if chemotherapy didn't help me before, why would it help me this time? My future seemed bleak.

"My thoughts then turned to Chi Lel. I had learned other types of qigong before but they didn't help. Would Chi Lel help? The only way to find out was to do it. So I told my husband that I was going to the Center.

"My husband, being a caring individual, said, 'It takes days by train to the Center and you are so weak. What if you die on the way there?'

"I replied, 'If I should die on the train, so be it, my husband.' My mind was made up that Chi Lel was my last hope. Once at the Center, I felt wonderful because I was no longer a patient! I worked assiduously and was amazed at my own ability to do so much exercise. What a sharp contrast to merely resting in bed, wishing my illness would go away. Meanwhile there was blood coming out in my urine. This lasted for two weeks."

"Did you call the doctor?"

"What doctor? I was my own doctor. If I was truly sick, how come I was so energetic and spirited? So I ignored the blood and continued to do what I was supposed to do—practice. Then my joints began to cause me a lot of pain. Still I wasn't worried by these chi-related symptoms and continued my practice. My strength returned to me each day I practiced. Within three months, the doctors couldn't see any cancer in my bladder."

"So you are cured?"

"At least the lumps are gone. I never take things for granted and I am still working as if I were fighting my enemy. It is a battle which will continue to the day I die."

"Why did Chi Lel help you but not other types of qigong?"

"In Chi Lel, we do it together to obtain a group-healing effect."

"Isn't it true that people do other qigong methods in groups too?"

"That's true, but even if you practice by yourself you can still experience a group effect if you can bring the group-healing chi your way. You must do this in order to truly know the difference. Simply practicing with others is not enough."

For Ms. Xiang, the difference meant life and death.

92. More Limber at Sixty Than She Was as a Girl

After giving a difficult birth to her son in 1956, Teacher Zhang's health went downhill. She had a kidney operation in which the wound didn't heal for a long time. Then in 1979 she had a high fever for a month, requiring hospitalization.

"Then three years later, the doctor told me that I had a tumor growing in my stomach and suggested an operation. The prospect of another operation frightened me because of my previous experience. Besides, I had cardiovascular problems which might trigger a heart attack during an operation. With nowhere to turn, I went to the park in search of something which might help me avoid surgery."

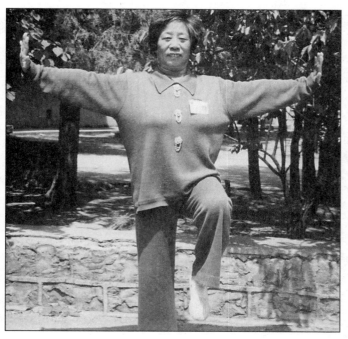

Zhang Fu-Di, 60, teacher

"Why to the park and not to another hospital?"

"I'd had enough hospitals. When I saw so many people practicing self-healing arts in the park, I began to wonder, 'Are these slow, meditative movements effective in healing oneself? If not, why are so many people practicing them every day? Are they all crazy?' Figuring I had nothing to lose, I made up my mind to try Chi Lel. It turned out to be the best decision I ever made in my life."

"Was it easy for you?"

"Not quite. I had to overcome the pain in my right shoulder, which had been immobilized for many years, and in my left leg, which was plagued with degenerative joint disease. Every time I went to group practice, I would walk painfully like I was rowing a boat. My body was squeezed to one side and I looked awful."

"Was your body in good shape before you were sick?"

"Yes, at least my husband had once told me that my body was gorgeous. When I got older, I was less concerned with my body shape than with being healthy. However, after three months of Chi-Lel practice, not only had my stomach tumor disappeared, but my body had returned to its original shape." With a smile, Teacher Zhang stood up and turned around.

"That's quite impressive, Teacher Zhang."

"Well, for a sixty-year-old woman, it's not too bad!" Then Teacher Zhang bent down to touch the ground with both her palms and said, "I couldn't do this before. Indeed, I am more limber today than when I was a little girl."

"So like ginger, the older the spicier?"

"I don't know about that. But I am becoming better every day."

"So in Chi Lel, the more one practices, the better one becomes?"

"I believe so."

93. Born In Hong Kong

Teacher Lin, who is in charge of a correspondence course for the Center, has a lot of connections to the outside world. She was born in Hong Kong and went to school in China during the war. Instead of returning home after graduation, she fell in love, married and settled down in China.

"During the Cultural Revolution, I was criticized and denounced as a Capitalist because I was from Hong Kong and one of my brothers was a university professor in the United States. The mental stress which accumulated during those years later manifested itself in physical illnesses.

"I had severe headaches, trigeminal neuralgia, pain in my spine, neck, and small intestine, a rapid heart rate, cancer in my reproductive organs, and Parkinson's Disease."

"Were you able to work all those years?"

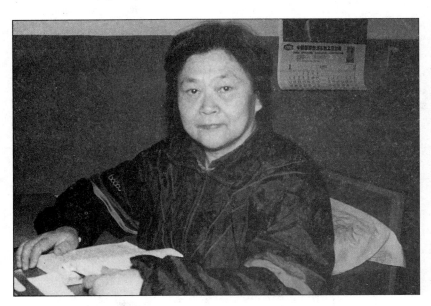

Lin Pei-Dan, 66, teacher

"Barely. Because of my analytical mind and a strong will to excel, I was able to overcome my physical pain. I jogged about twenty minutes a day while taking medicine to suppress my ailments. But when I discovered my body muscles quivering and my facial muscles becoming paralyzed, I began to look for other exercise methods. When I saw people practicing Chi Lel, I began to investigate."

"Investigate?"

"I mean I began to approach the subject as if I were doing a research project by reading many books and talking to different people. My final conclusion was that I should try it. So in 1981 I began my Chi Lel earnestly by practicing all day except during the time spent eating or sleeping."

"Why did you take it so seriously?"

"Through my investigation of Chi Lel, I became convinced that I could cure my own illnesses if I could work hard enough. Since I could do the movements all day long without exhaustion, I practiced on as if there were no tomorrow. As I practiced, I felt the changes in my body, which in turn motivated me to go on practicing until all my illnesses were gone."

"How long did it take you?"

"Half a year."

"Are you still practicing every day?"

"Every day, rain or shine—or snow. Of course, it only takes me about an hour now instead of the whole day."

"Excuse me Ms. Lin, but I noticed at times that your muscles still tremble a bit. Did you say you are cured?"

"You should have seen me fifteen years ago. Nerve diseases are supposed to become more severe as one ages. But now at the age of sixty-six, I can still work eight hours a day and take care of myself like anybody else. To me, this is a dream come true."

94. A Woman From Inner Mongolia

Born and raised in the grassland of Inner Mongolia, Ms. Liu has seen more cattle than people, and lived closer to nature than to the modern world. But diseases strike both city and country people alike.

Ms. Liu, like most people in villages, could tolerate her leg pain and stomachache. But when she was diagnosed as having kidney stones and an ovarian tumor, she couldn't ignore them even if she tried. Avoiding hospitals all her life, Ms. Liu was afraid of the smell of medicine and the sight of needles.

"Why were you afraid of going to the hospital?"

"The doctors put needles into my butt."

"They were helping you, weren't they?"

"I guess they were trying to. But my illnesses didn't go away. Then one day a friend told me about Chi Lel and I began the exercise two months ago."

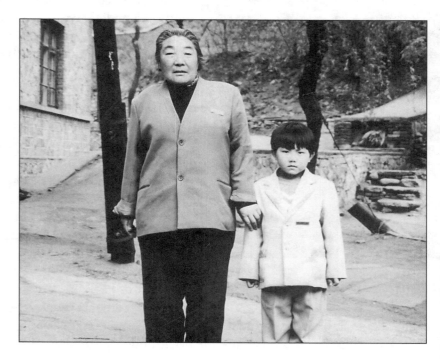

Liu Zheng-Chong, 68, student, with granddaughter

"How did your friend convince you to take Chi lel?"

"When my friend told me that Chi Lel was a natural healing method, I asked, 'No needles?'

'No needles.'

'No drugs?'

'No drugs.'

'Then it is for me. Where is the Center?' So I came here immediately. Once at the Center, I followed others exactly even though I didn't comprehend the chi theory."

"Have you ever questioned if Chi Lel would help you?"

"I had nothing to lose, why should I question this or that? I am only a simple old woman and I just follow what the teachers had told me."

"So your illnesses disappeared?"

"That's right. After two months' practice, the doctors put me in some kind of machine and told me that my diseases had vanished. Now I am as free and happy as the eagles over the grassland."

"What is your advice for others?"

"Keep it simple—just do it."

95. Taking Care of Daughter, Mother Was Healed

Like any concerned mother, Ms. Gao was worried when her daughter, who was a doctor trained in Western medicine, developed liver disease.

"Even though I myself had uterine fibrosis, I was too preoccupied with my daughter's illness to be concerned with my own condition. Even though the doctors couldn't help my daughter, I didn't give up hope and still tried to find a cure. When a neighbor told me about Chi Lel and its amazing effects, I immediately brought my daughter to the Center. When we arrived at the Center, I registered as a family nurse to my daughter, not as a student."

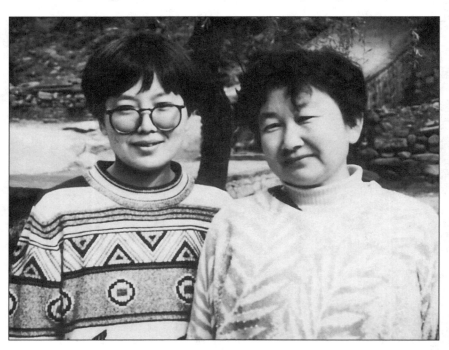

Gao Yu-Mei, 48, student, and her daughter

"Why?"

"I only wanted my daughter to get well. My heart ached as I watched her health deteriorate. Besides, we only wanted to try Chi Lel for a month. If it didn't work, we would move on to something else."

"Why?"

"Because my daughter's illness couldn't wait. But just after the first month, my daughter already felt better and we decided to stay on. Meanwhile I casually mentioned my illness to my daughter's teacher, who said to me, 'You are already here. Why don't you make the best of it?'

"Agreeing with the teacher, I decided to become a student. Like every student, I needed to get a diagnosis at the beginning of the treatment. After examining me by ultrasound, the doctor couldn't find anything wrong with my uterus. Indeed, my fibrosis had disappeared!"

"So by loving and caring for your daughter, you yourself were healed?"

"Yes. But while I was taking care of my daughter, I was also practicing Chi Lel."

"How did your healing affect your daughter?"

"My recovery gave my daughter a boost in her confidence also. Her condition has improved instead of deteriorating since we have been here. Now is our third month in the Center."

"How long will you stay here?"

"Until my daughter is healed."

"Can you afford the expense?"

"She spent more money in one month by herself in the hospital than we together will spend in one year at the Center. Of course, it won't take a year for her to recover."

Why was Ms. Gao so sure about her daughter's recovery? The answer was clear—she herself was living proof that the conventional way of treating a disease may not be the only way. What is incurable in one method of treatment may not be incurable in another.

96. I Feel As If I Were in My Thirties Again

Four years ago, Ms. Wang was hospitalized for three months after being diagnosed as diabetic.

"When doctors told me that there wasn't a cure for diabetes and that I would be on medication for the rest of my life, I asked heaven silently, Why me? Haven't I suffered enough? I was already afflicted with arthritis, and for fifteen years I had been weakened by a strange disease in which only half of my body could sweat."

"Did heaven hear your prayers?"

"It did. Soon a neighbor reminded me again of Chi Lel, which he had told me about a year ago. I jumped at the chance to learn this art."

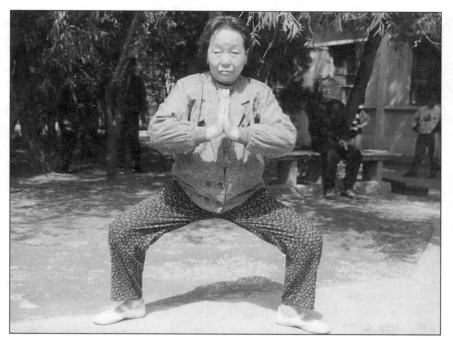

Wang Hung-Mei, 57, instructor trainee

"Why didn't you take up the art when your neighbor first mentioned Chi Lel to you? Didn't you believe in self-healing at the time?"

"I neither believed nor disbelieved but was only indifferent. As long as I could suppress my pain with medication, what was the point of exercising every day? If things aren't broken why fix them! But when doctors told me that my new illness would only become worse I began to have a different view. I was galvanized into action and joined my neighbor's Chi-Lel group.

"After twenty days of practice, I could walk, eat and sleep better. My spirits were high as I realized that my illness wasn't getting worse. Practicing diligently every day, I was able to gradually lessen the doses of my medications much like a baby being weaned off her mother's milk. But it took two years of practicing Chi Lel before I finally was totally independent of drugs. Now my diabetes and all other ailments have been cured for more than two years. Indeed, I feel as if I were in my thirties again."

"How so?"

"It was after that time in my life that I became sick and spiritless. The time in between my late thirties and early fifties were lost years—a true nightmare. Now in my late fifties, I can enjoy life as before."

"Has this nightmare made you appreciate life more?"

"Oh yes, I do love life very much, especially a healthy one!"

Being alive is a precious thing; being alive and healthy is even more precious.

97. Money Can Buy Surgery But Love Can Heal

Seven years ago when Ms. Deng first felt pain in her hips, doctors couldn't find anything wrong with her. But when the pain gradually went away, she was startled to find that her legs were shrinking.

"Then doctors X-rayed me and found that the blood supply to my femoral heads was cut off, resulting in femoral head necrosis. They told me that eventually I would need surgery if I wanted to walk again. Meanwhile my legs continued to shrink unevenly, resulting in my right leg being two inches shorter than my left."

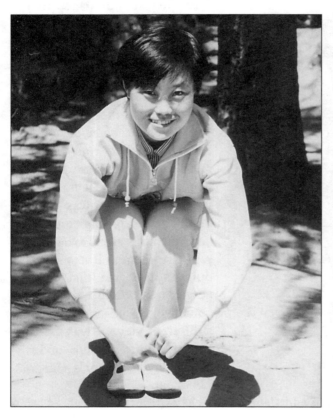

Deng Xue-Hua, 28, student

"Were you married then?"

"Yes, and I had one child. Even though my husband was a cheerful and understanding person, the prospect of a crippled wife hung like a shadow over our whole family. I dreaded the day when the inevitable would arrive and I would lose my ability to work in the field."

"Didn't the doctors say surgery would help?"

"Yes, they did, but everything costs money and surgery isn't cheap. We couldn't have afforded it even if it would have saved my ability to walk.

"Just when I thought my future was doomed, a distant relative told me about Chi Lel and encouraged me to try it. It was the first time that I was told there was hope for my hopeless situation. So I began to practice Chi lel, with a belief that even if it didn't heal my legs, it would generally improve my health.

"After a month's intensive training, I started to have feeling in my hips and I noticed that my right leg had grown longer! Now, after three months in the Center, my legs have returned to their original length and I can walk without bobbing up and down like I'm stepping into potholes with every step."

"Are you happy now?"

"Are you kidding? I am ecstatic!"

"Where do you want to go from here?"

"I am entering the Chi-Lel instructor's training program next month and I would love to be a teacher someday."

"They don't pay much for the Chi-Lel teachers. Do you know that?"

"Money is not everything but love is. Money can buy surgery but love can heal. Even without pay, I still want to be a teacher—to share with my students that I understand and love them just as much as my teachers loved and nurtured me."

"With what you have experienced, I am sure you will be an inspiring and loving teacher. Best wishes, Ms. Liu."

Indeed, love is a kind of powerful, healing chi within those who are willing to share it.

98. An Old Woman Shouldn't Go

Ms. Li had high blood pressure and coronary problems for years. Then in 1994 she was also diagnosed with diabetes.

"I had to stay in my house year-round because I was too weak to walk. The doctors told me that diabetes was a lifelong disease and that my family would need to take care of me. In fact, my daughter did become my around-the-clock nurse."

"It would have been long-term care since you were only fifty-five years old, wouldn't it?"

"No, it wouldn't have been too long. For me, I was already an old woman at fifty-five and ready to see the 'yin world.' When a neighbor advised me to go to the Chi-Lel Center, my daughter insisted that 'an old woman shouldn't go.' She was afraid I might lose my life by going on a long journey, but my husband encouraged me to go because by going to the Center, I would still have a thread of hope. Otherwise I would surely die a slow and painful death at home.

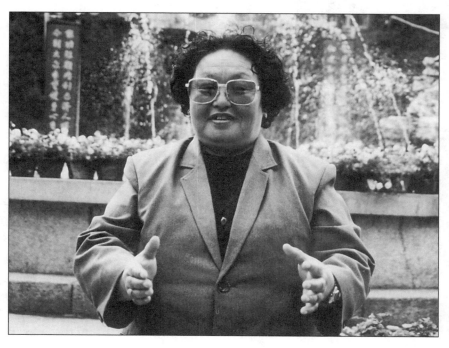

Li Sho-Sha, 56, student

"Once at the Center, I somehow felt released. After shaking hands with Lao-shi, I was healed. My blood sugar returned to normal and I could walk and run without chest pains."

"Ms. Li, are you telling me that you took medicine for a year for a severe case of diabetes and then became medicine free in less than two weeks?"

"Yes, that's what I saying."

"Some diabetic students take a much longer time to gain total recovery, how were you able to heal so quickly?"

"Lao-shi has said that some people heal almost instantly at the Center because the shape of their chi is identical to that of the chi field here. Therefore they can absorb healing chi without much difficulty. On the other hand, most people need much more effort to collect chi into their body for healing. I am one of the lucky ones."

"Does your daughter still call you an old woman?"

"No more. I hope one day she will call me big sister."

"Why?"

"By practicing Chi Lel, I feel and look younger every day. If she doesn't practice, I will eventually catch up with her in youthful looks!"

99. Sis, You Married the Right Guy

When Mr. Zhang was diagnosed with a liver tumor, doctors suggested immediate surgery.

"The doctors, in a fatherly tone, almost ordered me to undergo surgery because they thought it would be the best remedy for me. But I hesitated because I was afraid of the knife and pain. Besides, I had known people who had had surgery and still died. On the other hand, what would happen to me if my tumor was not removed surgically? Surely it would eventually grow so big that it would be beyond any help? It was just then, when I didn't know what to do, that my brother-in-law came to my rescue. He advised me to learn Chi Lel."

"Why did your brother-in-law suggest this alternative to you?"

"He had suffered for eight years with diabetes before being cured by Chi Lel. He was convinced that this self-healing art would help me too—but I wasn't so sure."

"Why not?"

"Well, I figured that even if Chi Lel was effective on diabetes it might not work for my disease. Unless it happened to me, I wouldn't truly believe it. But my brother-in-law insisted that I try. So with half-belief and half-doubt, I came to the Center. Once at the Center, I began practicing Chi Lel earnestly because I saw so many people with different illnesses being healed by these exercises.

"After two months of practice, I felt no more pain and could sleep and eat normally. The doctors confirmed with an ultrasound that my tumor was gone for good! What a relief!"

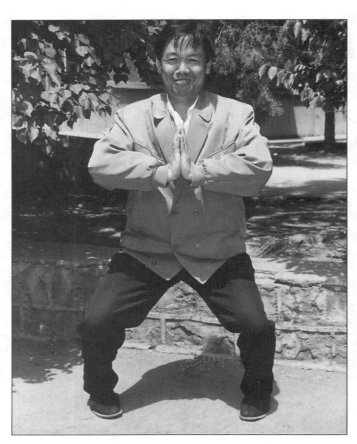

Zhang Men-Yu, 47, student

"Are you a believer now?"

"Of course, but sometimes I still think it is all a dream. Without medicine, without pain, it is just too good to be true. But when I do my Chi Lel everyday I understand that it is real—I feel the power of the universal chi inside and outside me."

"Now that you are well again, what will you say to your brother-in-law when you go home?"

"Well, I know what I will say to my sister: 'Sis, you married the right guy.'"

100. No More Needles

A year ago Mr. Liu began to feel weak, spiritless and thirsty all the time. When local doctors told him that he had incurable diabetes, Mr. Liu didn't believe them.

"At first, I didn't know what diabetes was and thought that if our local doctors couldn't cure my disease I should go to the best hospital in our country—the Beijing #301 Hospital. I figured

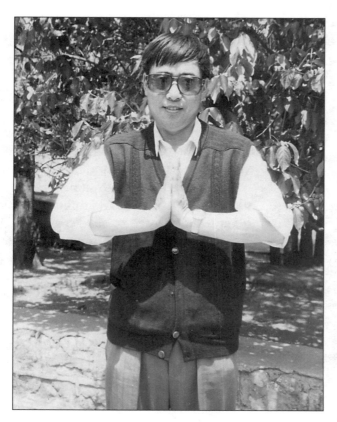

Liu Man-Shan, 38, student

that the big-city doctors there would surely have certain remedies which were inaccessible to small-town doctors. But when these prestigious doctors also prescribed the same medicine, insulin, for my illness, I was devastated. It was then that I truly believed that my illness was incurable.

"Once I realized that I would live with my ailment the rest of my life, I calmed down and faithfully injected my insulin every day. Oh, how I loathed those needles! But what could I do? However, when my brother advised me to try Chi Lel, I wasn't interested."

"Why not?"

"At the time I believed that if the doctors in the #301 Hospital couldn't heal my illness, who else could do it? If Chi Lel was so effective why hadn't the doctors mentioned it to me? After all, they were supposed to serve the people. So I dismissed my brother's advice as wishful thinking."

"So what changed your mind?"

"One day, after waking up in the morning, I stared at my lifeless face in the mirror and cried. My life was nothing but a syringe of insulin. Then I remembered my brother's words, 'Don't capitulate without a fight.' It was then that I decided to take up a self-healing art and fight the abnormality inside my body."

"So you abandoned your insulin immediately?"

"No, I got rid of it gradually. Once at the Center, I spent so much time doing Chi Lel that I didn't have time to dwell on my problem. Without thinking about it, my body gently healed itself as chi began working within me. After a month, doctors told me that my blood sugar was normal and there wasn't any sugar present in my urine."

"Are you still taking medicine now?"

"No, no more needles."

"Are you afraid that your illness might return?"

"No, as long as it is curable, what is the fear? Of course, I will keep on doing Chi Lel every day, not only to prevent the resurgence of my illness but to prevent other potentially life-threatening diseases as well."

With chi on his side, Mr. Liu is well equipped to fight any future illnesses.

101. An Eighty-Year-Old Educator

The smooth skin, steady gait, and alert mind of Mr. See indicated that he was no more than seventy years old. So I was quite surprised when Mr. See told me that he was actually eighty. And, when he handed me his business card, I was awed by his six impressive titles: he was a high government official.

"Because of my position in the government, I have access to our education secretary to persuade him to include Chi Lel in our school system. I believe if students can do Chi Lel every day as an exercise, it can increase their intelligence and strengthen their bodies."

"Why are you so convinced that Chi Lel would be beneficial to students?"

"We have done some experiments on school children in which results have shown that students, after doing Chi Lel for a period of time, have improved their grades."

"How did you get involved with Chi Lel?"

"When I was seventy, I was diagnosed with lymphoma. I could neither eat nor walk and, lying in bed, had to be fed through tubes. In the hospital, the doctors told me that I was too old to have chemotherapy and wanted to send me home immediately. But because of my connections, I was able to go through the back door to stay in the hospital for a longer time and get a second opinion. Unfortunately, I was again told that the side effects of chemotherapy would kill me if I had any more treatments. So, with this death sentence, I was sent home.

Shi Chung-Shu, 80, with wife

"While at home waiting to die, one of my subordinates suggested that I learn Chi Lel. Normally, I would have chastised my subordinate for believing in miracles, but in this extraordinary circumstance, with my illness eating me alive, I needed something to believe even if it was too good to be true. So I began my journey of self-healing, hoping to extend my life one day at a time. However, I got more than what I hoped for—I found a cure. Now at the age of eighty, I am still alive and well."

"What is your goal in life?"

"I am working very hard to persuade the government to include Chi Lel in school curriculums so that all the students in China can have an opportunity to learn Chi Lel."

"Do you think you will succeed?"

"I don't know. People, especially authority figures, are generally afraid of change, because new things bring new responsibilities and new responsibilities sprout new criticisms. However, I will continue to tell people the truth: that Chi Lel has healed me and that it holds great promise for improving the intelligence and health of mankind."

"With your position and prestige, I am sure that you have great influence."

"Everybody counts, and anyone healed by Chi Lel has influence. Eventually the number of us who have been cured will be so large that it will be impossible for the government to ignore us."

"Let's hope."

Part Two:

The Methods

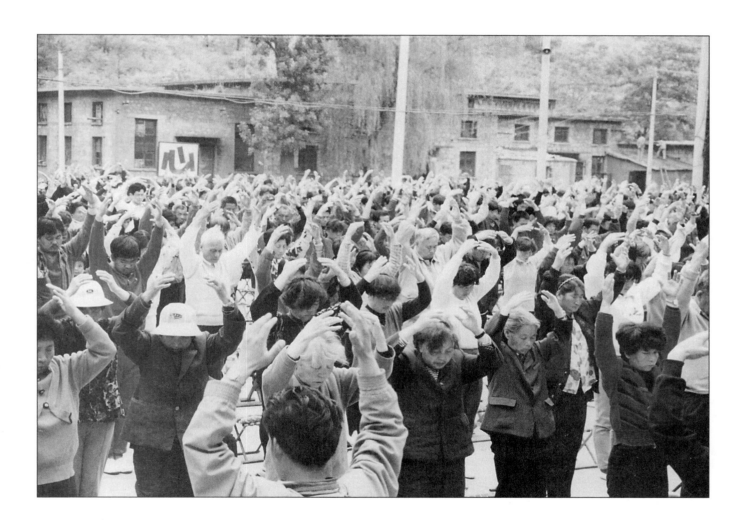

INTRODUCTION TO THE METHODS

After my article "The World's Largest Medicineless Hospital" was published in several magazines, I received many letters. One reader even faxed me an urgent message seeking my help in diagnosing his wife's illness because they were afraid of hospitals. I wrote to him immediately explaining that I am not a doctor and urged him to consult a physician without delay.

Was I being in contradictory to my own beliefs? No, because in health matters we must use the best available tools. Upon arrival at the Center, students are diagnosed with X-ray, CT, ultrasound, EKG, and other modern medical equipment. Chi diagnoses are simply not as reliable as machines. However, once a person has been diagnosed with a certain disease, it is then up to that person to make an informed decision as to how to deal with his or her own situation. If patients choose to undergo medical treatment, Chi-Lel exercise will aid their recovery or help them tolerate procedures like chemotherapy better. Even those who choose to do only Chi Lel, are still under the supervision of a doctor. For example, students at the Center are required to be diagnosed again after one month. Chi Lel should be treated not as a panacea, but as a scientific exercise. Illness is a serious matter and should not be put in blind trust.

Once a young man who was participating in one of my one-day Chi-Lel workshops in Cincinnati inquired, "I have diabetes. If I go to China, will they heal me?" For a moment I was

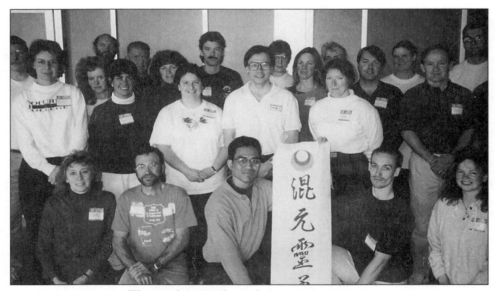

The author and workshop participants

at a loss for words. This young man had apparently been coerced by his father into taking my class because up to that point in the workshop he hadn't demonstrated any effort or interest in actively learning this self-healing art. Chi Lel is a "self-service" method. At self-service gas stations, once you've been shown how to use the gas pump, it's up to you to pump gas whenever your car runs low on fuel. If you don't want to pump gasoline into your car, how can you expect your car to run? Similarly, if this young man wasn't willing to practice Chi Lel, how would his

126

body return to normal? Chi Lel can't help those who won't help themselves, whether they are in the United States or in China.

On another occasion a participant in my workshop commented, "I have seen a qigong master who could move the hands of a person without even touching him—so powerful!" As she spoke she looked straight at me as if asking, "Can you also do this? Are you a true master?"

A person skilled in martial qigong may not be so adept at healing qigong and vice versa. When I interviewed students whose cancers had been dissolved by chi being emitted through their bodies, they told me that they hadn't felt any special sensation of chi when being treated. In other words, the healing chi from Chi-Lel teachers doesn't move the body, but rather penetrates it. In my workshops, I often emit chi for the healing of participants. Generally, chi works in such a subtle way that people just feel good and healing occurs without fanfare.

To the question of whether I am a true master or not, I frankly admit that I am not. That's why I still practice qigong diligently every day even after doing it for twenty-eight years. There's a story that once, when a student told his master excitedly that he had finally seen the light after so many years of meditation, his master replied calmly, "You will get over it, my student." Indeed, there is always a level above where one is now.

One day I received a call from a woman in Houston. After some pleasantries, she "pointed to the deer to curse the cow," asking, "I once knew someone who boasted about being a chi healer, but he later disappeared when he was revealed as a fake." I told her politely that I was not claiming any special powers and that I merely wished to introduce to the general public methods used by the largest qigong hospital in China.

How could I have defended Chi Lel over a long distance call? There are so many types of qigong in China that sometimes it is difficult even for experts to differentiate the "fish eyes from the real pearls." Some masters claim to have just come down from the mountains and are ready to save the world; some claim they bear the true lineage of some secret qigong; some claim to have obtained true transmission by divine intervention. They are all very appealing. In fact, at this time Chi Lel is not even the most popular qigong in China. From time to time, new types of qigong pop up and become overnight sensations. However, many of them eventually fade away.

Then why Chi Lel? I chose Chi Lel primarily for two reasons. First, Chi Lel is reliable because it has been practiced daily by millions of people for many years. Would you rather trust an automobile which has shown no defects after being driven by millions of people under all kinds of conditions for many years? Or would you rather venture out to try something new?

Second, Chi Lel is a scientific and progressive self-healing system that utilizes the world's largest medicineless hospital for research and training. The system was developed by a respected grandmaster, Dr. Pang, who understands medicine and is not afraid to combine modern medical technology with traditional qigong. Under Dr. Pang's guidance, the Center has been a leader in developing new healing techniques which, like new generations of computers, work faster and more efficiently than their predecessors. Indeed, Chi Lel is on the leading edge of chi therapy.

Some time ago a radio-talk-show host, a qigong practitioner, remarked, "It took me years to learn qigong. How can you teach Chi Lel to people in just a few hours?" I told him that many of the students coming to the Center are dying, and therefore don't have years to learn. So the method has to be simple and to the point. Indeed, in just a few hours Chi-Lel students can learn the movements and then follow audiotapes, just as people in aerobics classes follow audiotapes, and derive benefits immediately from the first workout.

Then why, in the old days, did students take years to learn qigong? For one thing, the masters were testing the loyalty of their students; for another, it was a good way of learning. Imagine following a master for a number of years and then suddenly one day he invites you to his inner room and whispers to you, "Think blue sky when you are doing the opening movements and the inside of your body when you are doing the closing movements." You listen intently as your master's words penetrate deep into your mind. After so many years, now you have finally obtained the secret and you will practice, practice, practice until you master it. On the other hand, if your teacher tells you during the first lesson that the secret of Chi Lel is to alternately think of infinity and then the inner body, you probably will take his words lightly and not practice the art seriously and end up with nothing.

Dr. Pang has revealed his qigong secrets to you and you can learn them in a few hours. It's up to you to take them seriously or not. As a consequence of the revealing of qigong secrets, the traditional master-student relationship no longer exists. I often tell my workshop participants that I am not their master and that my job is nothing other than to present in its entirety the Chi-Lel method which is taught in the Center.

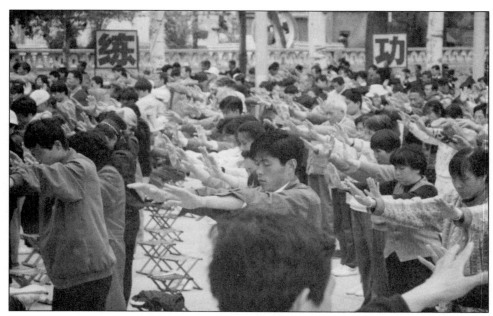

Students practicing Chi Lel at the Center

Another frequently asked question is about breathing in Chi Lel. Because the Chinese character for chi is closely related to the character for air, many people mistakenly believe that qigong is about breathing. However, air and chi are not the same. In Chi Lel, we emphasize normal breathing. When you're relaxed, your breathing is natural, slow, deep, and gentle. You don't need to deliberately think about the breathing process. Indeed, not only your lungs, but your entire body breathes when you practice Chi Lel.

According to Dr. Pang, there are many types of chi. In Chi Lel, we use *Wan-yan chi*, the finest chi in nature. Wan-yan chi, the building block of everything, is a colorless, shapeless thing which fills the whole universe. Our body is made up of Wan-yan chi, called Inner Chi; and the immediate space around our body is also filled with Wan-yan chi, called Outer Chi. There are constant exchanges of Inner Chi and Outer Chi through our pores and the pressure points along our meridian systems. In practicing Chi Lel, we amplify this natural exchange process by directing our thoughts first to infinity and then back to our body.

By opening our body to the universe, we are dissolving the blockages so that chi can flow vigorously through our body, bringing life energy to every cell. Without blockages, we become balanced, healthy, happy, and full of energy and vitality, not just free of illnesses.

Qigong is a generic name for any method which involves the exercise of chi. The Chinese spell the word "chi" as "qi". Because English-speaking people cannot pronounce "qigong", sometimes "chigong" or "chi-kung" are used instead. Dr. Pang's qigong system, called Zhineng Qigong (zhineng means intelligence), consists of many levels. The Center prescribes the first level of Zhineng Qigong, which consists of the *Lift Chi Up and Pour Chi Down* and *Three Centers Merge Standing* methods, for their students. For simplicity and differentiation from other qigong methods, we call it Chi Lel. So when we say we are practicing Chi Lel, in essence we are saying that we are practicing Zhineng Qigong as it is taught in the world's largest medicineless hospital.

Chi Lel has four main components:

1. Belief (*Shan Shin*): While belief is not a must for people to receive chi healing, as shown by babies who couldn't have believed in chi and yet recovered, it is nonetheless a very important part of self-healing. Experience at the Center tells us that only a small percentage of people can readily absorb chi, so most people will require persistence to achieve the benefits of Chi Lel.

Imagine you are thirsty and someone tells you that there is water in the ground one hundred feet beneath you. You then begin to dig a well, but, like anything else worthwhile, your progress is slow, say only one foot a day. After a few days you begin to doubt whether there really is water underneath you. Meanwhile hundreds of other things scramble for your attention and you quit, saying, "There is no water down there."

But wait, there is water down there and you can find it if you would just keep on digging every day for one hundred days. Do you believe the statements of the 101 individuals interviewed in this book? They are the testimonials of those who have found water. Have faith, keep on digging, and the water will be there. This is the power of belief.

2. Organization of a Chi-field (*Chu-Chong*): While at the Center, I taught English to one of the teachers. During our first lesson, my student surprised me by saying, "Wait, let's form a chi-field." We closed our eyes and she gathered Wan-yan chi from infinity, forming a chi-field which would facilitate learning. With her thinking harmonized with mine and the whole universe, she quickly learned what I had to teach.

Organizing a chi-field, Chu-Chong, means the leader of a group harmonizes the thinking of the members of a group for learning or healing. First, the leader surveys the group with his eyes, forming a boundary around the group; he then verbally relaxes the group's members from head to toe; then he directs the group to alternately think of blue sky and then their bodies, bringing down Wan-yan chi from the sky to form a huge energy field, surrounding everyone in the group.

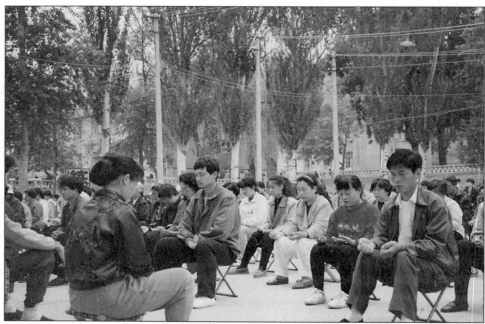

Students organizing a chi-field

In a group setting, the power of chi is multiplied because of the aggregate effect of the individual chi-fields of the people in the group, just as a group of people, each carrying a candle, will brighten up the whole room. The larger the group the more powerful the chi field, and so also the healing effect.

What if you practice alone at home, do you still need to organize a chi-field? Yes, you need to form a chi-field between yourself and the universe. In this sense you are not alone: millions of Chi-Lel practitioners around the world are forming chi-fields every day and as a result, the whole world is shrouded in a huge Wan-yan chi-field. Moreover, every full moon the founder, Dr. Pang, organizes a chi-field for all Chi-Lel practitioners in the world. In United States, the time is 8:00 P.M., E.S.T. every full moon. So let's practice Chi Lel together! Wherever you are, join with us.

3. Facilitating chi for healing (*Fa-Chi-Gee-Ping*): How is it that chi can heal? If you could see the videotape footage I took in China of bladder cancer being dissolved by chi in real time, would you say it's unbelievable? Not if you understand the behavior of chi. For thousands of years the Chinese have consistently affirmed that when chi gathers matter appears and when chi disperses matter dissolves. According to Dr. Pang, Wan-yan chi, although powerful, listens to our command. So this cancer, which had appeared as matter when chi gathered in an unbalanced way, disappeared without a trace when Chi-Lel teachers emitted chi into it, rearranging abnormal chi into normal chi.

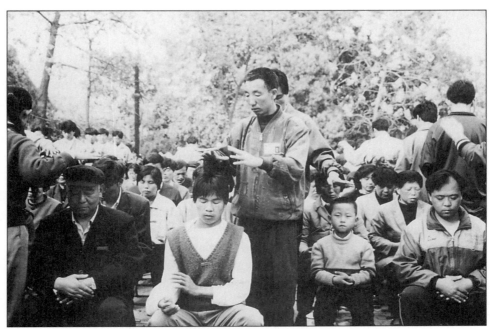

Teachers emitting chi to students

At the Center, to illustrate "chi gathers—matter appears," they restore a cracked egg by emitting chi to it. Amazingly, it returns to its original, unbroken state. I was told that there have been many incidents of broken bones being healed instantly by Chi-Lel teachers commanding chi to gather where bones had been broken.

How do you facilitate chi for healing? You use the technique known as *Chu-Chong-Gee-Ping*: organizing a chi-field for healing. First you organize a chi-field and imagine all the persons in your group joining into one being. Then you direct chi, which is already gathering, into this being by saying aloud phrases such as "chi and blood are plentiful," "meridians open," "illness disappears," "body functions return to normal.," and "*Hou La* (cured, healed, recovered)."

In traditional Chinese medicine, it is believed that chi and blood are closely related and their abundance is essential for vigorous health. Therefore we suggest to our bodies that chi and blood are plentiful. Moreover, because chi flows through meridians, we suggest that our meridians are open so that abundant amounts of chi can flow through us unimpeded.

Even when facilitating chi healing for only one person, you still need to organize a chi-field as you would do for a group. Please remember that you are not emitting your own chi to the other person, but rather you are facilitating for healing the chi in the chi-field of the being which was formed during the organizing of the chi-field. It is very important for you to include yourself in this being so that while you are facilitating chi flow to others you are also absorbing chi. While healing others, observe the subtle distinction between using your own chi and the universal chi.

How to protect yourself from giving your chi away? Practice. Actually when you are practicing Chi Lel, you need to use the same process for organizing chi-field as you would for a group, except in this case, you facilitate chi for your own healing. The more you practice, the more you will able to facilitate the chi in the universe, instead of your own chi, for healing others and yourself.

4. Practice (*Lan-Gong*): To obtain the benefits of Chi Lel, there is no substitution for practice. If someone emits chi to you and you feel good today, unless you begin to practice Chi Lel, by tomorrow you will have lost this good feeling, just as if someone gives you a bowl of rice today, tomorrow you will again be hungry.

Only through hard work can one truly master the art of qigong. For thousands of years, China has never found a "Mozart" in qigong. If someone claims that he can open your meridians for a large fee, ask him, "If this is so, why don't you open your sons and daughters' channels so that they, too, can be masters like yourself?"

Gong is a principle which states that accomplishments are the result of a long period of daily effort. Let me define gong more simply: one hundred days of consecutive practice. So if you can practice Chi Lel consecutively for one hundred days, you have accomplished one gong. Consecutive practicing means that if you miss one day, you need to start all over again. For beginners, fifteen minutes a day keeps the doctor away. Sound simple? Until you try it! One practitioner told me that he had to start all over again because he had fallen asleep on the ninety-fifth day; another one told me that several times she had gotten up in the middle of the night to do Chi Lel because she had forgotten to do it during the day.

As you begin to feel more comfortable with the routines, you may want to increase your practice to thirty minutes or more. Do it with an audiotape because it will help you to concentrate. If at first you have a feeling of chi but lose that feeling after practicing Chi Lel for sometime, you may be going through a period of growth. Why? Because as a beginner you are like a small container which quickly fills with chi. Then as you practice you become a bigger container. Your chi is not yet sufficient to fill up this larger container; therefore you will not feel anything until you fill it up and are again ready to go on to another level.

Is morning or evening better for practicing Chi Lel? Both, if you can practice twice a day, because the more you practice, the better the results. But if you can only practice once a day, choose a time which is best for you and stick to it even if you are on an out-of-town trip. And, though you don't need to face any particular direction when practicing Chi Lel, choose a spot in your home and practice in that same place every day. When you practice Chi Lel in the same room for some time, a chi-field is formed. People in this room will feel good even though they don't practice Chi Lel. One practitioner told me that her husband's illness had shown improvement since she began Chi Lel. Another practitioner told me that her cat sat next to her every time she practiced Chi Lel; another reported that her plants had grown more luxuriant and had flowered longer and better. This is no surprise, since it is the power of chi that gives energy to our lives. Chi is within all of us, and it is now up to you to discover it.

1. Lift Chi Up and Pour Chi Down Method (*Pun-chi-kwun-din-fa*)

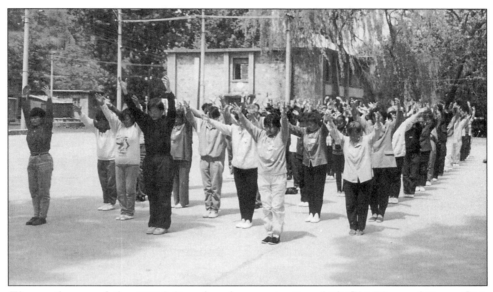

The author and the 101 Miracles demonstrating Lift Chi Up and Pour Chi Down Method at the Center

This is the main method practiced by students at the Chi-Lel Center. For beginning students, the exercise takes about fifteen minutes. For other students, the movements are slowed down to thirty minutes. Depending on your needs, you can repeat the routine many times. The more you practice, the better the results.

A. Characteristics of *Lift Chi Up and Pour Chi Down Method*:

1. Exchanging Wan-yan chi: When doing the opening movements, you release your Wan-yan chi to infinity; when doing the closing movements, you absorb Wan-yan chi from nature. By collecting and exchanging chi with nature, your meridian system is opened. Years are added to the lives of those whose chi flows uninterrupted.

2. Strong feelings of chi: After practicing for a relatively short period of time, you will begin to feel chi. When chi arrives, your illnesses disappear and your energy level is increased.

3. Developing sensitivity: After practicing for awhile, your body becomes more soft and sensitive and your mind becomes more aware of natural things such as flowers, trees, mountains, rivers, lakes, rain, thunderstorms, sun, moon, and stars.

4. Developing the ability to facilitate chi for healing: Daily practice allows you to quickly master the technique of facilitating chi for healing others without depleting your own chi.

5. Visualizing the movements being done in infinity: You use your mind intent (yi) to attract chi by imagining you have become an infinitely large being, with your head touching the sky and feet deeply rooted in the earth. Every opening and closing movement occurs on the horizon. By opening up, you can become one with nature. In this natural state, you are vigorously healthy and infinitely joyful.

Here are eight sentences designed to help practitioners enter into a qigong state:

1. "Head touches sky, feet stand on earth (*Ding-ten-lee-dee*)": Imagine your head reaching to the sky and your feet deeply rooted in the earth. Since the earth is suspended in space, you can now imagine your feet blended into the earth and your body suspended in space.

2. "Body relaxes, mind expands (*Shing-shung-yi-chung*)": Relax your entire body from head to toe and from inside to outside. Then imagine the front, back, left, and right sides of your body expanding to the horizon. Now you are the only person occupying the universe. You and nature have become one.

3. "Be respectful and quiet (*Why-chin-nine-ching*)": By doing Chi Lel, you are embarking on a journey of self-discovery. This is a respectful endeavor. Being respectful of what you do will enable your mind to calm down. When your mind is quiet, you will be able to enter into a qigong state.

4. "Mind is clear and appearance is humble (*Shin-ching-mau-kung*)": When your mind has quieted down and become clear, it will, like the smooth surface of a natural pond, reflect yourself. As you show respect to Chi Lel, your appearance will be humble.

5. "No distracting thoughts (*Yee-nan-bu-chee*)": Empty yourself of all thoughts.

6. "Think space (*Shen-chu-tai-kung*)": Even though you don't have any thoughts, your mind intent is in space, in infinity.

7. "Think body (*Shen-yi-chia-te*)": Bring the mind intent back from infinity to your body.

8. "Entire body is harmonized with chi (*Chow-shin-yo-yo*)": As the mind intent returns to your body it brings back Wan-yan chi from infinity. As your body is suffused with chi, you enter into a comfortable and blissful state of qigong.

134

Preparation for *Lift Chi Up and Pour Chi Down Method**:

1. Stand straight with feet together, body centered, hands hanging naturally next to your thighs. Look at the horizon and then slowly withdraw your vision inward and gently close your eyelids (Fig. 1).

2. Meditate on the following eight phrases: Head touches sky, feet stand on earth; Body relaxes, mind expands; Be respectful and quiet; Mind is clear and appearance is humble; No distracting thoughts; Think space; Think body; Entire body is harmonized with chi.

I. Commencing Sequence:

1. With little fingers leading, rotate your hands sideways and then down until your fingers point forward and palms face the ground. Using your shoulders as pivots, push hands forward fifteen degrees (about one palm's length) from your body; imagine the centers of your palms connecting to earth chi. Then pull your hands to the sides, next to thighs, to collect chi. Repeat this push and pull for a total of three times (Fig. 2,3,4).

2. With little fingers leading, relax your wrists and turn palms to face each other, with *Tiger Mouth* (area between the thumb and index finger) facing upward. Relaxing your shoulders, move your hands up, shoulder-width apart, lifting chi, to the navel level. Slightly cup palms and reflect chi to navel (Fig 5). Turn palms down and visualize your arms reaching to infinity. With your hands at infinity, move them behind you at navel level to your back. Withdraw your forearms a little to turn palms inward; then slightly cup palms to reflect chi to *Mingmen* (pressure point on spine directly opposite navel, refer to Pressure Point Diagram on page 151). Move your hands upward and forward to beneath armpits, and use the tips of middle fingers to pour chi into *Dabao* (pressure point along the spleen meridian, between the sixth and seventh ribs, Fig. 6, 7, 8).

3. Extend your hands forward with palms up to shoulder level and width. Move middle fingers toward forehead to reflect chi to *Yintang* (area between eyebrows, Fig. 9, 10). At the same time, turn wrists slightly until hands face each other diagonally; then, leading with elbows, separate your hands and move arms to the sides, palms up, to form a straight line (Fig.11). With little fingers leading, turn your palms down, and then up, imagining your hands extending to the horizon. With your hands at the horizon, lift them up along the blue sky to above your head. Bring your hands together (Fig.12,13,14). Then lower your hands to chest level, forming a praying position (forearms creating a straight line with middle fingers pointing up and thumbs about one-fist distance from body, Fig. 15).

*Demonstrated by Pan Hung M.D. (Interview 2).

II. Commencing from Front and Lifting Chi from Side:

1. Point your fingers forward and extend your hands forward at shoulder level (Fig. 16, 17). With thumbs and index fingers still touching, gradually open your hands so the palms face down. Raise palms, then slowly separate fingers and move arms apart to shoulder width. Now fingers should be pointing up, and hands perpendicular to arms (Fig. 18, 19). Imagine your hands extending to the horizon; keeping them at the horizon, push and pull three times to collect chi. Shoulders, elbows, and wrists move in unison with shoulders moving up, back, down, and forward in a circle. When pulling, move your shoulders upward and backward. At the same time, slightly drop your elbows, cup palms, and think body; returning your mind from the horizon. When doing the pushing, move your shoulders down and forward leading with the bottoms of the palms, and visualize your hands reaching the horizon (Fig. 20, 21). With palms extending to the horizon, open and close three times to collect chi horizontally. Open your hands about fifteen degrees (about one palm's length), to the sides and close hands to shoulder width (Fig. 22, 23).

2. With fingers pointing up, circle your arms to the sides, forming a straight line (Fig. 24). Visualize your hands extending to the horizon, and keeping them at the horizon, push and pull three times to collect chi. When pulling, move your shoulders up and inwards. At the same time, slightly drop your elbows, cup palms, and think body; returning your mind from the horizon (Fig. 25, 26). When pushing, move your shoulders down and forward, leading with the bottoms of the palms and visualizing your hands reaching the horizon. With palms extending to the horizon, move your hands up and down three times to collect chi vertically. Move your hands up about fifteen degrees (about one palm's length) and back to shoulder level (Fig. 27, 28).

3. Relax your wrists and turn the palms upward. Visualize your hands reaching to the horizon; keeping them there, lift chi up to above your head with arms slightly bent and wrists above your shoulders. Then slightly cup your palms to reflect chi to the top of your head. Pause for a moment (about one cycle of breath) while pouring chi into your body through the top of your head (Fig. 29, 30). Lower your hands along the body centerline, moving hands in front of your face and then to the chest. At chest level, turn your palms in and continue to lower hands to navel. Press navel with the middle fingers (Fig. 31, 32).

4. Circle hands around your waist, imagining fingertips touching inside your body to Mingmen, and then press Mingmen with your middle fingers (mind intent reaches navel). Move your hands down along hips, thighs, calves, and ankles, imagining your hands combing inside your legs (Fig. 33, 34). Circle your hands around your feet and place your hands on top of them (fingers and toes point in the same direction). Press down and move up three times to collect chi. When pressing, kneel forward, shifting your body weight forward to the hands (mind intent penetrates through the centers of your palms and feet into the earth). When moving up, lift your knees and move your buttocks up and backwards (mind intent moves from the earth back to the body) with hands remaining in contact with feet (Fig. 35, 36). Then lift your hands slightly and turn them to face each other as if holding a balloon, using your mind to extract chi from earth. Separate your hands and turn the palms to face your inner legs. Raise your hands along the calves, knees, inner

thighs, abdomen, and navel (Fig. 37, 38, 39, 40). Press navel with the middle fingers. Separating your hands to the sides, return to the beginning position (Fig. 41).

III. Commencing from Sides and Lifting Chi in Front:

1. Slowly raise your hands from the sides with the palms down, forming a straight line (Fig. 42). Raise palms. Visualize your hands extending to the horizon, and keeping them at the horizon, push and pull three times to collect chi (Fig. 43, 44, 45). When pulling, move shoulders up and inwards. At the same time, slightly drop your elbows, cup palms, and think body; returning your mind's intent from the horizon. When pushing, move your shoulders down and forward, leading with the bottoms of your palms and visualizing your hands reaching the horizon. With palms extending to the horizon, close and open your hands three times to collect chi horizontally. Close your hands about fifteen degrees (about one palm's length) forward and open them to form a straight line (Fig. 46, 47).

2. With fingers pointing up, move your hands forward along the horizon to shoulder level and width. Keeping your hands at the horizon, push and pull three times to collect chi. Shoulders, elbows, and wrists move in unison with shoulders moving up, back, down, forward in a circle. When pulling, move your shoulders up and backwards. At the same time, slightly drop your elbows, cup your palms, and think body; returning your mind intent from the horizon. When pushing, move your shoulders down and forward, leading with the bottoms of your palms and visualizing your hands reaching the horizon (Fig. 48, 49, 50). With palms extending to the horizon, move your hands up and down three times to collect chi vertically. Move your hands upward about fifteen degrees (about one palm's length) and back to shoulder level (Fig. 51, 52).

3. Relax your wrists and turn the palms up. Visualize your hands reaching the horizon; keeping them at the horizon, lift chi up to above your head with arms slightly bent and wrists above your shoulders. Then slightly cup your palms to reflect chi to the top of your head. Pause for a moment (about one cycle of breath) while pouring chi into your body through the top of your head (Fig. 53, 54). Lower your hands along the body centerline, moving them in front of your head to Yintang. Press Yintang with your middle fingers (Fig. 55). Circle your hands around your head, along the eyebrows, to Yuzheng (the pressure point located opposite Yintang) and press Yuzheng with the middle fingers (Fig. 56). Direct your fingers down along your neck and spine to the third thoracic vertebra. Press this vertebra with the middle fingers, elbows facing sky (Fig 57). Then move your hands over shoulders and under armpits to reach up as far as you can along your spine to connect chi. With palms close to body, lower your hands to Mingmen and press Mingmen with your middle fingers (Fig. 58, 59).

4. Circle hands around your waist, imagining fingertips touching inside your body, to navel and then press navel with your middle fingers (mind intent reaches Mingmen). Move hands down along your abdomen, thighs, knees, calves, and ankles, imagining hands combing the inside of your legs (Fig. 60, 61). Place your hands on top of feet (fingers and toes point in the same

direction). Press down and move up three times to collect chi. When pressing, kneel forward, shifting your body weight forward to the hands (mind intent penetrates through the centers of your palms and feet into earth). When moving up, lift knees and move your buttocks up and backwards (mind's intent moves from the earth back to the body), with hands remaining in contact with feet (Fig. 62, 63). Then lift your hands slightly and turn them to face each other as if holding a balloon, using your mind intent to extract chi from the earth. Circle your hands backwards to the back of the ankles. Raise your hands along the calves, thighs, and hips, to Mingmen and press Mingmen with middle fingers (Fig. 64, 65, 66). Circle your hands around waist to navel and press it with your middle fingers. Separating your hands to the sides, return to the beginning position (Fig. 67, 68).

IV. Commencing from Diagonals to Lift Chi:

1. As if holding an object, raise your arms, with Tiger Mouth (the space between your thumb and index finger) facing upward, at forty-five degree angles with the direction you are facing. Your arms will form a ninety-degree angle with each other (Fig. 69). When your hands reach the shoulder level, turn the palms up and continue to raise your hands. Meanwhile, visualizing your hands reaching the horizon and staying there, lift chi up to above your head, with your arms slightly bent and wrists above the shoulders. Then slightly cup your palms to reflect chi to the top of your head. Pause for a moment (about one cycle of breath) while pouring chi into your body through the top of your head (Fig. 70). Lower your hands along the body centerline and then along your ears to the shoulders. Drop your elbows and turn palms forward with forearms in front of your shoulders and perpendicular to the ground (Fig. 71, 72).

V. Return Chi:

1. Drop your right wrist and push right arm forward (Fig. 73) until it's almost straight. Relax wrist and, with little finger leading, turn your palm to the left (Fig. 74). Moving from the waist, scoop chi to the left. When your body has turned ninety degrees, press *Zhongkui* (pressure point located in the second segment of middle finger, Fig. 75) with your thumb; slightly closing fingers, continue to move your hand around shoulder almost 180 degrees. Return your body to the front and, with thumb still pressing Zhongkui, press left-shoulder *Chihu* (located underneath collar bone and above nipple) with the tip of your right middle finger. Pour chi into Chihu (Fig. 76).

2. Drop your left wrist and push left arm forward until it's almost straight; relax wrist and turn your palm to the right. Moving from the waist, scoop chi to the right. When your body has turned ninety degrees, press Zhongkui with your thumb; slightly closing your fingers, continue to move your hand around shoulder almost 180 degrees. Return your body to the front, and, with thumb still pressing Zhongkui, press right-shoulder Chihu with left middle finger. Pour chi into Chihu.

3. Your arms now cross each other in front of your chest, forming a forty-five-degree angle with the body (Fig. 77). Breathe naturally three times; press Chihu with your middle fingers while breathing in and release your fingers while breathing out. Then separate fingers and push hands forward, turning the wrists to form a Lotus Palm. Close your hands to a praying position in front of your chest (Fig. 78, 79).

VI. Closing Sequence:

Raise hands in front of your body to above your head. Raise hands slightly more, imagining you are touching the sky (Fig. 80). Separate your hands and turn the palms forward. Lower your hands to the sides, forming a straight line. Turn palms up and, along the horizon, move your arms forward to shoulder width. Reflect chi to Yintang with middle fingers (Fig. 81, 82). Bring arms in towards your body and under arms (Fig. 83); press Dabao with your middle fingers to deliver chi, imagining fingertips are touching inside your body (Fig. 84). Stretch your hands backward (Fig. 85). Circle arms forward to the sides, turn palms forward and then close your arms in front of you, embracing chi (Fig. 86). Stack centers of your palms on navel (male left hand, female right hand first). Calm and nourish chi (Fig. 87). Separate your hands to the sides, returning to their original positions. Open your eyes slowly (Fig. 88, 89).

Figures shown on pages 140-144.

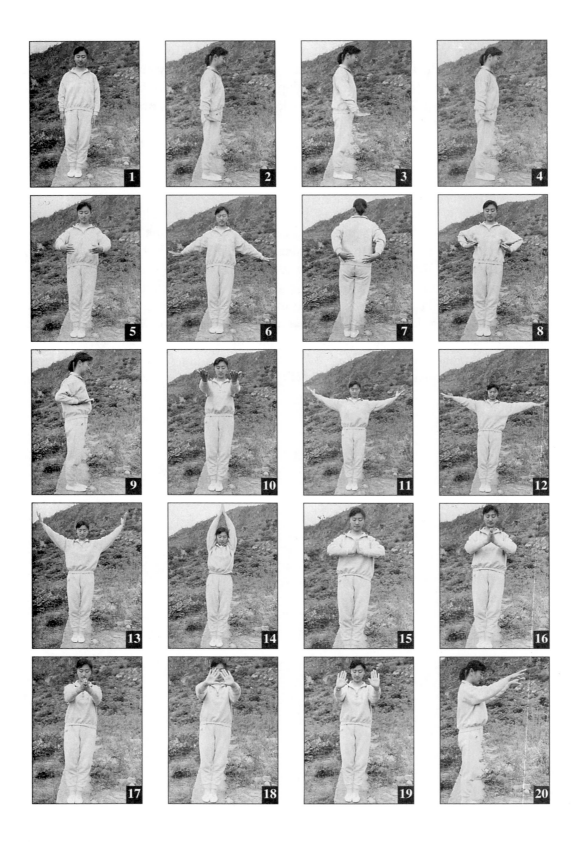

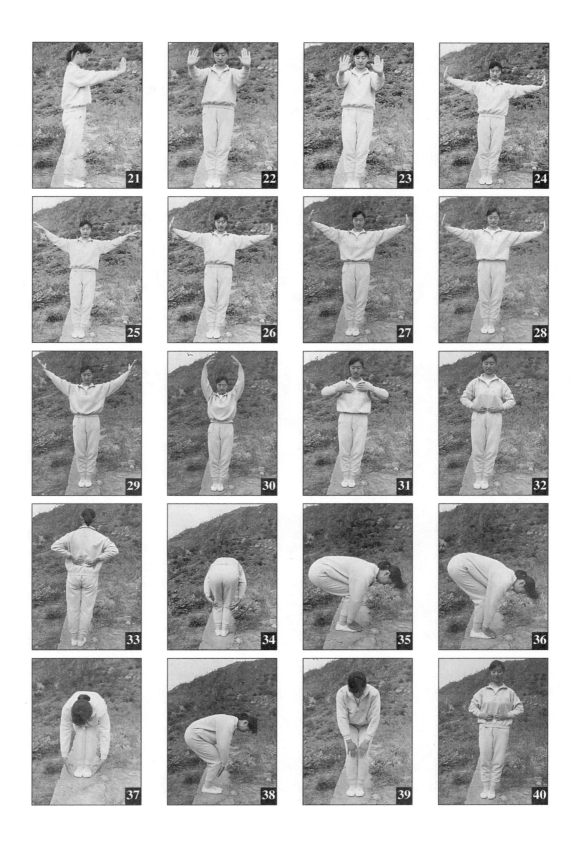

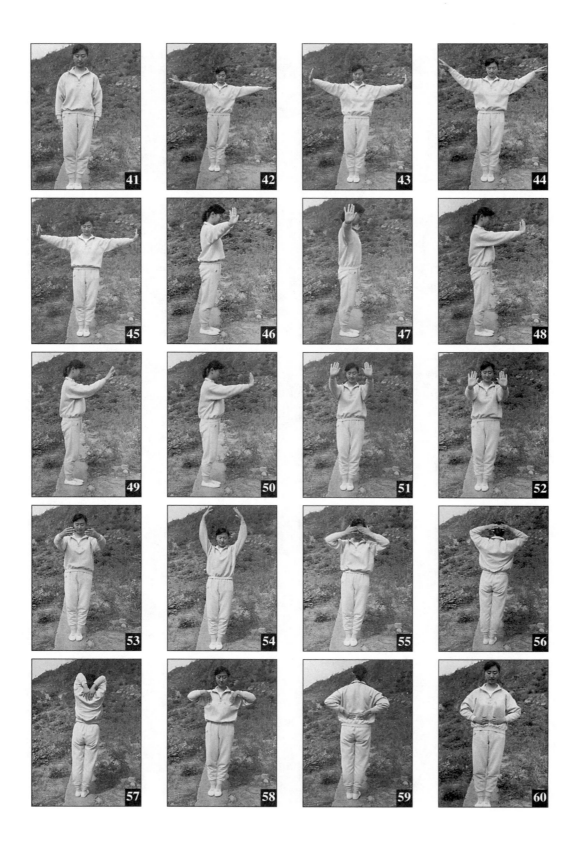

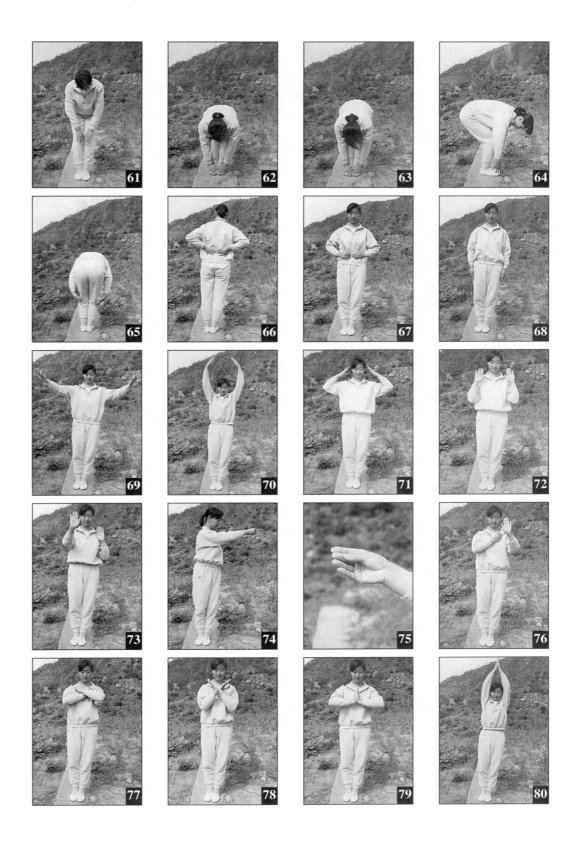

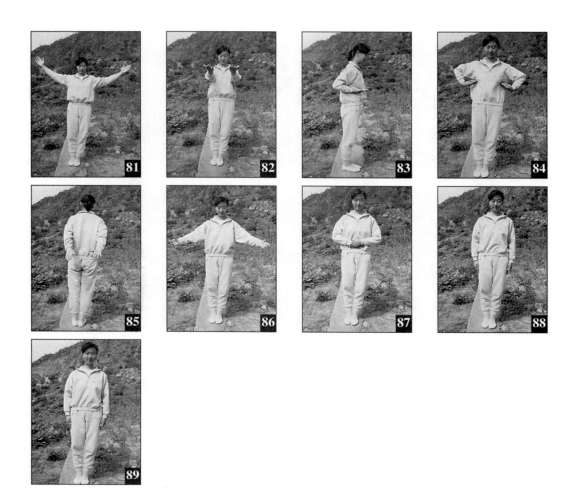

2. Three Centers Merge Standing Method *(Shan-Sin-Ping-Chon-Chong)*

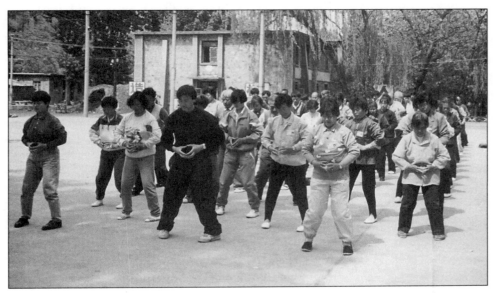

The author and the 101 Miracles demonstrating Three Centers Merge Standing Method at the Center

This is a stationary exercise in which one stands meditatively for about a half-hour at a time. By focusing on the *Dantian* (abdominal area between navel and Mingmen), you can quickly experience special feelings, such as warmth, in the Dantian area. It is an excellent way to loosen your hips and waist so that chi can circulate through the meridians uninterrupted. This method is not only good for health, it is also a fundamental training exercise for martial artists.

The commencing and the closing sequences of this standing method are the same as those in *Lift Chi Up and Pour Chi Down Method* except in the beginning where you stand with your feet apart.

1. Stand straight with your feet together, body centered, hands hanging naturally next to your thighs. Look at the horizon and then slowly withdraw your vision inward and gently close your eyelids.

Step on chi: Keeping your heels stationary, separate the front parts of your feet to form a ninety degree angle; then, with toes in place, separate your heels to somewhat wider than shoulder width (Fig. A1, A2).

2. With little fingers leading, rotate your hands sideways and then down until your fingers point forward and palms face the ground. Using shoulders as pivots, push hands forward fifteen degrees (about one palm's length) from your body; imagine the centers of your palms connecting to earth chi. Then pull your hands to the sides, next to thighs, to collect chi. Repeat this push and pull for a total of three times (Fig. A3, A4, A5).

3. With little fingers leading, relax wrists and turn your palms to face each other, with *Tiger Mouth* (area between the thumb and index finger) facing upward. Relaxing shoulders, move your hands up, shoulder-width apart, lifting chi, to the navel level. Slightly cup palms and reflect chi to navel (Fig. A6). Turn palms down and visualize your arms reaching to infinity. With your hands at infinity, move them behind you at navel level to the back. Withdraw your forearms a little to turn palms inward; then slightly cup palms to reflect chi to *Mingmen* (pressure point on spine directly opposite navel, Fig. A7, A8). Move your hands upward and forward to beneath your armpits, and use the tips of middle fingers to pour chi into *Dabao* (pressure point along the spleen meridian, between the sixth and seventh ribs, Fig. A9).

4. Extend your hands forward with palms up to shoulder level and width. Move middle fingers toward forehead to reflect chi to *Yintang* (area between eyebrows, Fig. A10). At the same time, turn wrists slightly until hands face each other diagonally; then, leading with elbows, separate your hands and move your arms to the sides, palms up, to form a straight line (Fig. A11). With little fingers leading, turn your palms down, and then up, imagining your hands extending to the horizon. With hands at the horizon, lift them up along the blue sky to above your head. Bring your hands together (Fig. A12, A13). Then lower your hands to chest level, forming a praying position (forearms creating a straight line with middle fingers pointing up and thumbs about one-fist distance from body, Fig. A14).

5. Slowly lower your hands to navel and at the same time gradually separate your palms, with fingertips slightly touching, as if holding a ball. Rest hands lightly on your abdomen with palms facing the navel. Slowly lower body as far as you can and still feel comfortable, with the knees not extending over the toes (Fig. A15, A16, A17).

Keep your feet on the ground without exerting much force on either side of the soles. Keep your knees relaxed and pointing inward slightly. Raise *Huiyin* (groin area); keep the inner thigh area round and relaxed, not tightly squeezed. Relax your abdominal area and waist, and keep the Mingmen area outward so that the lower back is round. Keep your tailbone perpendicular to the center of the iso-triangle formed by the heels and the back. You'll feel like you're sitting down yet you're not sitting. Relax your shoulders and drop your elbows, but keep the armpits open. Relax your wrists and cup your palms.

Suspend your head as if its being pulled from above. Hollow your chest, not by collapsing the shoulders but by relaxing the chest muscles. Raise your back to straighten the spine. The purpose of hollowing the chest and raising the back is to increase lung capacity while relaxing the chest and back.

Relax the area between the eyebrows, keep your tongue touching the upper palate, relax your facial muscles and keep a joyful face as if smiling.

6. Closing Sequence

Slowly straighten your legs and, stepping on chi (i.e., keeping the bottoms of both feet on the ground), bring your feet together by first rotating heels and then toes. Slowly raise your hands while closing fingers to form a praying position in front of chest (Fig. A18, A19). Raise your hands in front of your body to above the head. Raise hands slightly further, imagining they are touching the sky (refer to *Lift Chi Up* Fig. 80 to Fig. 87). Separate your hands and turn the palms forward. Lower your hands to the sides, forming a straight line. Turn the palms up and move your arms forward to shoulder width; middle fingers reflect chi on Yintang. Bring your arms in towards body and under arms; press Dabao with your middle finger to pour chi in, imagining fingertips are touching inside your body. Then stretch your hands backward. Circle your arms forward to the sides, turn palms forward and then close arms forward embracing chi. Stack the centers of your palms on navel (male left hand, female right hand first).

Massage your abdomen, circling nine times in each direction, first counter-clockwise and then clockwise. Calm and nourish chi. Separate your hands to the sides, returning to their original positions. Open your eyes slowly.

Figures shown on page 148.

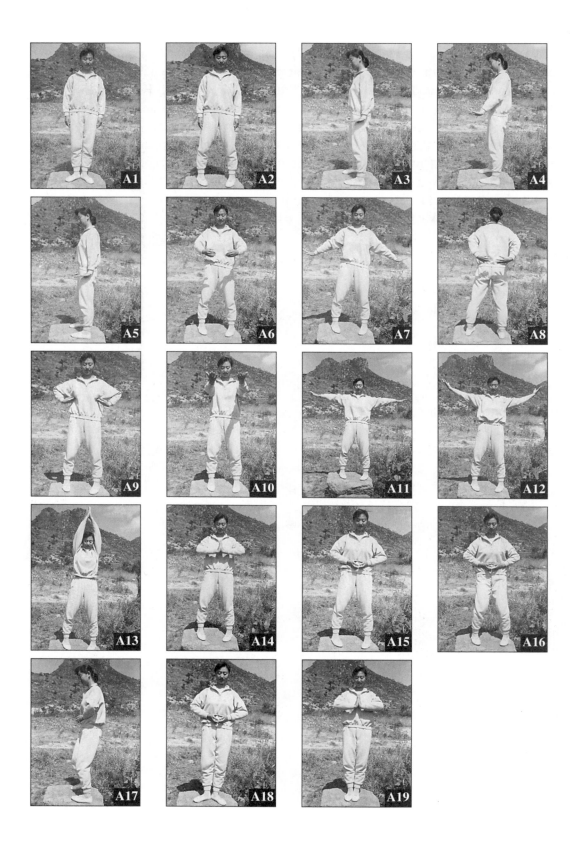

148

3. Wall Squatting*

Wall Squatting, *Ton Chong*, although a simple exercise, was a well-kept secret for generations. It is an effective way of loosening up your waist and stimulating chi flow throughout the body.

Just as the name Wall Squatting suggests, this exercise is done by moving up and down in front of a wall. With your nose, forehead, and feet close to a smooth wall, slowly squat down, relaxing your chest and hollowing in your shoulders (Fig. B1). When your thighs reach ninety degrees (Fig. B2), relax your waist with Mingmen going outward and continue to squat down until your thighs touch your calves (Fig. B3). Then move up slowly, with your nose and forehead still close to the wall (Fig. B4). When going up, think that the top of your head is being pulled up; when squatting down, think about relaxing the Dantian area. Repeat this exercise one hundred times per day for a hundred days or more.

For beginners, keep your feet apart or stand away from the wall and replace a wall with a pole, a tree, or something to hold on to if you lose your balance. Depending on your physical condition, you may want to begin with ten or twenty repetitions a day and gradually build to a hundred or even more.

Young students practicing Wall Squatting

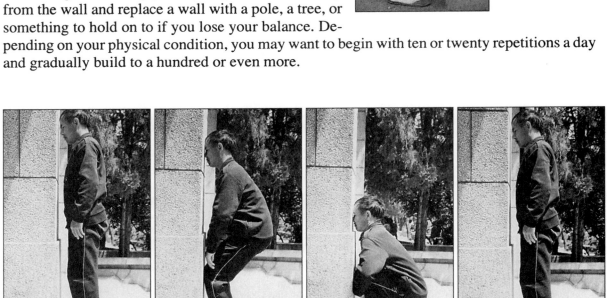

B1 B2 B3 B4

* Demonstrated by Teacher Jing (Interview 35)

4. La Chi*

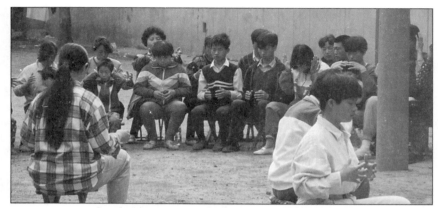

Students practicing La Chi at the Center

La Chi is simple and effective way of collecting chi for healing oneself and others. Many people in the previous interviews achieved amazing healing results by using this technique.

Put your hands close to each other so that fingers and palms almost touch each other (Fig. C1, C2). Relaxing your shoulders and hands, slowly open your hands to the sides (Fig. C3, C4). Then close your hands until the palms and fingers almost touch. Repeat these opening and closing movements many times. Very soon you will feel some sensations between your hands. These sensations are caused by chi gathering from the universe. Then deliver this chi into where is needed in your body. For instance if you have a headache, deliver chi into your head by doing the opening and closing movements near your head.

When doing the opening movement, imagine that your illness disappears into infinity; when doing the closing movement, imagine that you are delivering life energy into where it is needed. Meanwhile, suggest to yourself that chi is healing you and that you have recovered.

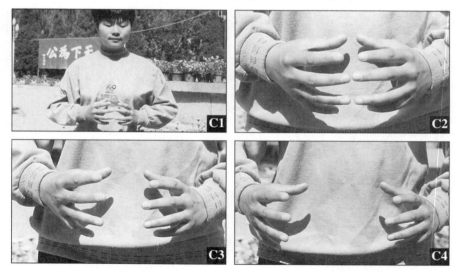

*Demonstrated by Teacher Liu (Interview 3)

150

Pressure Point Diagram

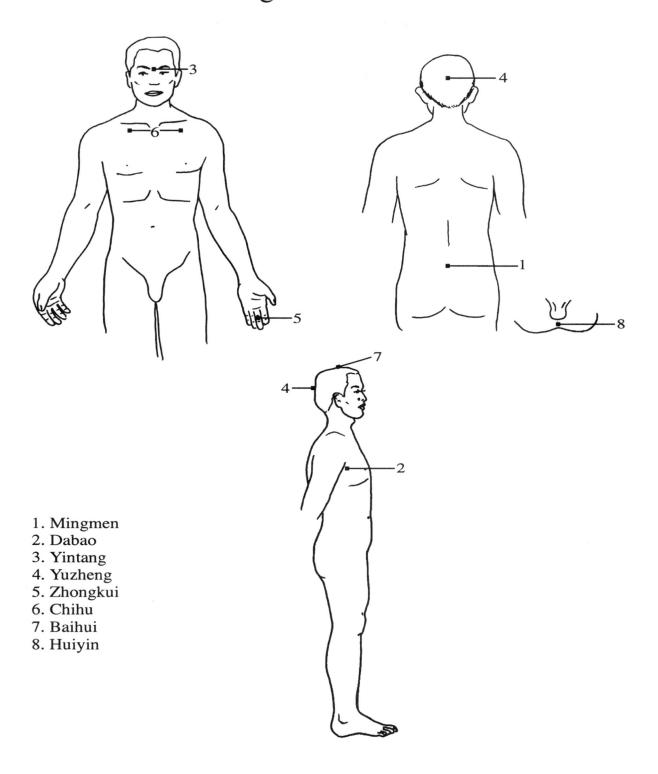

1. Mingmen
2. Dabao
3. Yintang
4. Yuzheng
5. Zhongkui
6. Chihu
7. Baihui
8. Huiyin

151

Chi Lel in America

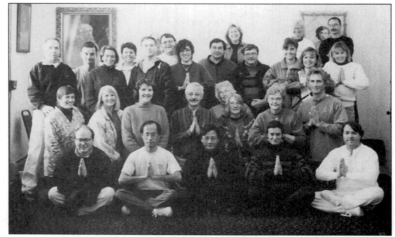

The author and his brother Frank Chan pose with participants in the first instructor-training retreat, 1995, Lily Dale, New York.

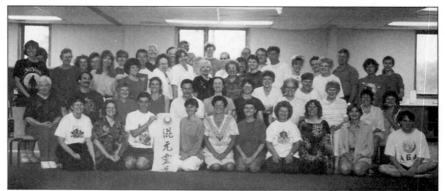

The author and participants in a workshop, Columbus, Ohio.

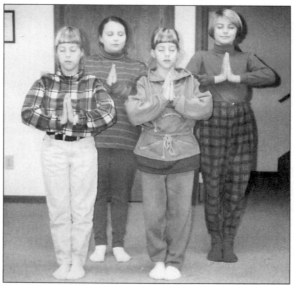

Twins Melissa and Megan (front), the youngest Americans(10-years old) to complete the100-day Lift Chi Up Method.

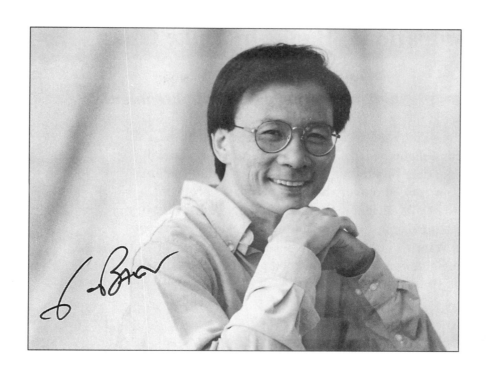

From the Author to the Readers:

☞ *If you would like to receive*

☐ **A free copy of our Chi-Lel newsletter**
☐ **My workshop and retreat schedules**
☐ **Information on Chi-Lel instructor certification programs**
☐ **Dates for trips to the Chi-Lel Center in China**

✍ *please wirte to or call me:*

Luke Chan
9676 Cinti-Columbus Road
Cincinnati, Oh 45241

513 777-0588 Fax 513 755-5722

Other Inspirational Books by Luke Chan

Secrets of the Tai Chi Circle: Journey to Enlightenment

Follow the journey of the student as he learns the Secrets of the Tai Chi Circle from his enlightened Tai Chi Grandmaster, and you will find all of us, at one time or another, haunted by yesterday's failures, worried about tomorrow, and overwhelmed by today's problems. But the gentleness of this ancient story, like a mighty boat, will carry you safely through the deepest gorges and the darkest valleys in your river of emotions. You will cry and you will laugh. Finally when you come out into the light, you will be a changed person. The joy of being alive will be yours *now and forever*.

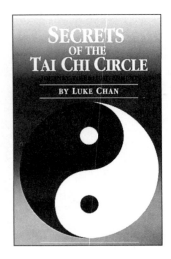

***Secrets* is available both in printed and audio versions.**

101 Lessons of Tao

These ancient stories of Tao will cause you to both laugh and learn. Reading each story is like looking into a still pond, with one aspect of your life reflected back to you. By recognizing the yins and yangs of your life, you can achieve a balanced state of Tao for optimal living. By knowing that others share your behavior, you can prevent yourself from feeling isolated and taking things too personally, thereby increasing your self-esteem and morale.

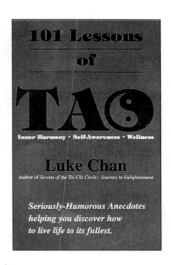

Accompanying Videotape and Audiotapes

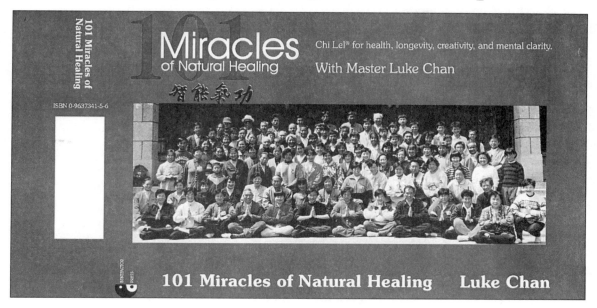

Videotape: 101 Miracles of Natural Healing
Chi Lel® for health, longevity, creativity, and mental clarity.

With Master Luke Chan

This videotape offers one hour and forty minutes of :
Step-by-step Instructions for—
  1. Lift Chi Up and Pour Chi Down Method.
  2. Three Centers Merge Standing Method.
  3. La Chi.
  4. Wall Squatting.
Actual Footage from China of—
  1. A bladder cancer being removed in real-time using chi.
  2. Testimonials of recovered patients.
  3. Group practice of Chi Lel.
  4. Fa Chi—emitting chi for healing from:
      a. Teachers to students.
      b. Family members to their loved ones.
      c. Founder, Dr. Pang, to students.

ORDER FORM

Videotape:
101 Miracles of Natural Healing $39.95 $ _____

Audiotapes:
1. *Lift Chi Up and Pour Chi Down Method* $10.00 $ _____
   Side A: 16 minutes
   Side B: 30 minutes with Founder's voice
2. *Advanced Lift Chi Up and Pour Chi Down* $10.00 $ _____
   Side A: 40 minutes
   Side B: 40 minutes
3. *Three Centers Merge Standing Method* $10.00 $ _____

101 Lessons of Tao:
Number of books _____ x $ 12.95 $ _____

Secrets of the Tai Chi Circle: Journey to Enlightenment
Number of books _____ x $ 10.00 $ _____
Audiotapes (4 pieces) _____ x $ 24.95 $ _____
Unabridged recording of *Secrets*

Postage and handling
($3.00 for first item, .50 for each add.) $ _____

Ohio residents add 5.5% sales tax $ _____

Total Amount Due $ _____

To order, please fill out this coupon and send with check or money order to:
   Benefactor Press
   9676 Cinti-Columbus Road
   Cincinnati, Oh 45241
   Tel 513 777-0588 Fax 513 755-5722

Name:_____

Address:_____

City:_____State:_____ Zip:_____

Visa Or Master Card Orders: 1-800 484-6814 Code 4264

Please allow 1-3 weeks for delivery. Thank You.